A Physician's Guide to Herbal Wellness

Safe and Effective Remedies for Achieving and Maintaining Health

John Cammarata, M.D.

Chicago Review Press

Library of Congress Cataloging-in-Publication Data

Cammarata, John.
 A physician's guide to herbal wellness : safe and effective remedies for
achieving and maintaining health / John Cammarata. — 1st. ed.
  p. cm.
 Includes bibliographical references.
 ISBN 1-55652-273-8 (pbk.)
 1. Herbs—Therapeutic use. I. Title
RM666.H33C363 1996
615'.321—dc20   96-12822
                                                                  CIP

©1996 by John Cammarata, M.D.
All rights reserved
First edition
Published by Chicago Review Press, Incorporated
814 North Franklin Street
Chicago, Illinois 60610

ISBN 1–55652–273–8
Printed in the United States of America
5 4 3 2 1

1996

A Physician's Guide to Herbal Wellness

*To those whose unfailing love, acceptance,
and forgiveness heal me daily—my parents, Marge and Tony,
my children, Aaron and Joel, and my wife, Kathleen.*

ACKNOWLEDGMENTS

Thanks to my father, who worked tirelessly and without complaint typing the original manuscript. Thanks to my son Aaron, the computer whiz, who spent many a long night working with me and without whose help the book would still be hopelessly locked in a word processor. Thanks to my wife, Kathleen, whose careful reading, ideas, and suggestions improved every page.

Thanks to Linda Matthews, Amy Teschner, and everyone at Chicago Review Press for their hard work and their tolerance toward a nervous and probably occasionally annoying first-time author. Thanks to Christine Adamek, who smoothed out the rough edges. And thanks to my agent, Bill Adler, Jr., who believed in this book from the beginning.

Lastly, a special thanks to my patients. I hope we can continue to educate each other about health and wellness for many years to come.

CONTENTS

PART 3

PART 4

CAUTIONARY NOTE

As you read through this book, please keep in mind one very important point: it is very dangerous to rely solely on herbs in maintaining good health. If you feel ill—for example, if you have chest pains—be sure to call your doctor. It's better to talk to or see your physician and learn that the problem is minor than it is to do nothing, relying solely on your herbs, as your condition becomes increasingly serious.

Also, don't count on a "quick fix" and expect that herbs will provide instant relief or a total cure for your medical problems. Although sometimes you'll see results within a week or two of taking a botanical, in other cases it may take as long as three to six months of regular use to see maximum benefits. Why? Because some herbs build up in the system, and the cumulative effect is what gives you the best results.

I believe that the proper use of herbs can enable many people to achieve a good level of wellness. But I also believe that you should keep your physician informed about what herbs you are using and why you are using them. (See the sections on "Herbalism and Your Physician" and "What if My Doctor Thinks Herbalism Is Weird? Or I'm Afraid He Will," in Chapter 1.) When in doubt, contact your doctor. Not your friends or relatives, but your doctor.

A Physician's Guide to Herbal Wellness was written to supply essential information and to educate the interested reader on the complementary nature of herbal and modern medicine. It is not intended as a replacement for medical advice, which should always be obtained through consultation with a health professional.

For the purposes of this book, herbs taken as separate substances but used at the same time as other herbs are considered to be a mixture. They need not be physically combined to be considered a formula or prescription.

I have used the words "drugs," "herbs," "medicines," and "medications" interchangeably.

INTRODUCTION

*F*or thousands of years, people have been using herbs success-fully to treat a wide variety of ailments. Interest in using this ancient knowledge is rapidly escalating today, as we realize that expensive prescribed medications are not always the one true path to take. Herbs may be used in combination with conventional medical treatment to help a person feel healthy.

But until recently, most physicians as well as the general public believed that using herbs was a sort of latter-day flower child 1960s thing to do. Probably not dangerous, but silly.

Botanicals (herbs) are not silly at all and can provide dramatic improvements to health, even above what standard medications can achieve, and often without the distressing side effects of many prescribed drugs. At the same time, however, although they are "natural," botanicals can be dangerous when taken to excess, as is also true of virtually every other substance.

Now many people are turning to herbal treatment. Experts report that sales of herbs in 1994 exceeded $1.6 billion in the United States, and sales continue to grow. (This amount doesn't include sales to Canadians, who are also intensely interested in botanicals.) Experts say that herb sales are projected to increase by up to 15 percent per year.

In most cases, botanicals are far less costly than are prescription medications, and you do not have to see a physician to purchase them. Instead, you go to a pharmacy or health food store—and in some cases, your local supermarket—to buy them.

In addition to this very high level of consumer interest and the overall low cost of herbs, another key factor is expected to further increase the sale of botanicals. The passage of the Dietary Supplement Health and Education Act of 1994 in the United States will enable those who market botanicals as beneficial foods to provide more consumer information than in past years and thus to heighten consumer interest and awareness. This act defined a "dietary supplement" as a vitamin, mineral, herb, amino acid, or other product and requires the government to prove a product unsafe. Of course, sellers may not make unreasonable claims, such as that a product cures AIDS or cancer, but they can make general health claims. This law is expected to be fully implemented sometime in 1997.

Consumer Knowledge Is Important

Consumers should be aware of the curative properties attributable to individual herbs and know, for example, which herbs are most likely to provide relief for specific ailments. *A Physician's Guide to Herbal Wellness* deals primarily with herbs and their medicinal properties. It provides necessary information for a careful use of herbs in human illness and is a practical book that can be referred to frequently.

A Physician's Guide to Herbal Wellness also gives readers important information to enable them to become more proactive and involved in their own health care, which is increasingly important today with "managed care" and other constraints. In addition, it's a very good idea for patients to be educated and aware in all areas of health.

While modern science has provided numerous effective medicines to combat disease, alternative medicine has given us the great legacy of its own philosophy. We each, individually, can increase wellness, prevent disease, and foster vitality. We, rather than the "doctor as god," are largely responsible for the state of our own health.

Said the great healer Paracelsus, "The physician is only the servant of nature, not her master. Therefore it behooves medicine to follow the will of nature." As we each assume a greater responsibility for our own well-being we should all pay heed to this wisdom.

Why I Wrote This Book

My path to medicine was typical for many physicians: biology major in college and then medical school—where you eat, drink, and sleep the science of human health and disease—followed by years of postgraduate training in a medical specialty (internal medicine in my case). Many years of study and application have convinced me of the validity and value of the scientific approach in healing patients.

My interest in botanicals grew out of a very distressing personal experience. In 1992 I had a heart attack, and during my recuperation I was put on various medications that caused me to feel lethargic and sleepy; I found myself going to bed as soon as I came home from work. I also suffered from painful swelling in my ankles.

I began to wonder whether there was some other way to achieve the same benefits without the side effects. Then over the course of eight months I underwent four angioplasties and ultimately had triple coronary bypass surgery. This is when I resolved to learn everything possible about herbal therapy. I began using botanicals myself and have continued to use them—and feel great!

Next I decided to use herbal treatments with some of my patients, with excellent results, particularly with arthritis, high blood pressure, and also with AIDS. (More information on my treatments is provided later in this book.)

Today I run a weight control facility and manage a clinic for drug addicts. I don't use herbs with my overweight patients, instead choosing pharmaceuticals. But I began to obtain very good results by recommending botanicals for patients with other ailments.

Patients were pleased and almost all felt they had benefited from herbal therapy. New patients began calling the office specifically for herbal consultations, and my practice developed a whole different dimension. It's been very personally fulfilling to me to see how well a carefully formulated herbal mixture compares with prescription medications. In my experience, patient satisfaction with herbal therapy is at least equal to that achieved with conventional medications.

Herbalism versus Modern Medicine

There was a leap of faith in this process of educating myself on herbs, because of the philosophical differences between herbalists and most physicians. I quickly became firmly convinced of the effectiveness and validity of herbal treatment, but fitting this herbal knowledge into a deeply ingrained perspective of modern Western medicine today truly required an open mind.

So I read further and learned more about the philosophy and worldview underlying herbalism. I came to appreciate that herbalism and modern medicine are not mutually exclusive and contradictory but instead simply represent different perspectives. I found that I needed to reconcile a cluster of seemingly disparate notions— health and disease, the ancient and the modern, art and science, and the physical and the spiritual—into an encompassing viewpoint.

One problem with medicine as practiced today is that too often it is a rigorous discipline based upon dispassionate science and hard cold facts, not taking individual needs into account. It has yielded remarkable breakthroughs, yet many people feel that a high price has been paid. Conversely, herbal medicine and other forms of alternative medicine are instead based more in the realm of experience and feelings and are adapted to the individual's personal needs. In this book I have attempted to be fair to both viewpoints to achieve an overall balanced outlook.

Another difference between herbalists and medical doctors is that herbalists believe that virtually everyone can benefit from using herbs and thus usage need not be limited to people who feel sick. Instead, they see people as evolving toward a state of wellness and see herbs as one means to improve daily health. In addition, they (and I) believe that if the herbs that are right for a person are used on a daily basis, then that person is likely to have fewer episodes of even mild illnesses.

In contrast, many medical doctors see patients only when they are ill, and the doctor's goal is to eradicate the illness—or, in the case of a chronic illness, to provide improvements. Thus the person is either "sick" or "well," and generally physicians do not see patients as on a continuum moving toward wellness. It's important to understand this philosophical difference.

Medical doctors may also distrust herbalists and patients using herbs because in most cases, neither herbalist nor patient has received a medical degree, and doctors worry that such ignorance could be dangerous. And yet it is also true that many medical doctors are completely ignorant of some very useful herbal treatments that would be less costly and more efficacious than the standard medication that is usually prescribed.

While some illnesses are better treated by modern medicine, others mandate the opposite. Many fall somewhere between these extremes; thus the individual could benefit from either modern medicine or herbal therapy. However, the major premise of this book is that the "either/or" choice is a false one. Instead I prefer a "both" approach. If I persuade you to share in my beliefs, then you'll agree that any health care system, to be complete, must embrace both. At bottom, they are complementary to each other, and I believe both are needed to form a whole system. I think it is a mistake to rely on only one when medical benefits can clearly be gained from each.

Although there are extremists in both the modern medicine and herbalist camps decrying the shortcomings of the other's approach, the truth is that the major differences in the two systems are more in emphasis than in substance. In both approaches, for example, an illness requires both treatment and recuperation for cure. One key difference, however, is that modern medicine, awed by the power of its ministrations, glorifies treatment. Herbalist medicine, more respectful of the human body and the toll that illness can take, gives the recuperation of the human body far greater emphasis. The important point is that there is little in either system that truly contradicts the other.

The goal should be to take what is of value in each system and apply it judiciously to the problems of combating disease and maintaining health. I believe that a coalition between health care systems is what is called for; the problems after all are universal and affect all humankind. We need to recognize that illness is the common enemy and that modern medicine and herbal medicine are each frameworks with valuable insights and remedies.

A Complementary Approach

We live in a time when there are many more questions than answers, especially when it comes to matters of health, illness, and personal well-being. The whole concept of amalgamating ancient and modern medical wisdom is in its infancy, although interest is rapidly growing among the general public as well as among many physicians. Reserved and halting steps, however, are preferable to none at all, and it is in this spirit that this book is presented.

The entire movement toward herbal wellness and complementary systems of healing represents a grassroots effort, and patients lead the way. The United States, Canada, and other developed societies are now questioning the most basic premises of modern medicine. And while politicians and the insurance industries endlessly debate the delivery of health care, many people are unsure of the type of health care they want delivered.

One thing patients do know is that they are far less willing these days to accept impersonal care; multimillion-dollar, high-tech machinery; and mutilating surgery as the only options for wellness. While we respect and often marvel at the successes our doctors have achieved, a simpler, more basic outlook toward health has also evolved.

Validating interest in the medical knowledge of past years, the National Institutes of Health (NIH) has created a Section on Alternative Medicine. It is charged with the responsibility of studying untested therapies, including herbalism. And the NIH is not alone.

Some of the most respected American medical schools, including the oldest, Columbia University's College of Physicians and Surgeons, now offer courses in alternative medicine—or what we have learned from the past, as opposed to our high-tech approach today. Scholars from all medical disciplines debate the value of herbal therapy and acupuncture. Meetings for M.D.'s are now devoted to these previously taboo topics, and I see this as a very positive and enlightened step up to where we need to be.

With the passage of sufficient time, as well as a willingness to learn and a sense of fairness accompanied by a requisite degree of humility, fundamental changes can occur. I believe that the scientific and alternative healers who currently view each other with suspicion and distrust will then see each other as partners with different approaches and taking different roads, but also with the ultimate goal of reaching the same destination: the wellness of patients.

The Meaning of Complementary Medicine

Implicit in the very word "complementary" is the notion of incompleteness. When two things complement each other they together form a whole and require each other for sufficiency.

When we apply the complementary idea to medicine today, we might compare it to a marriage between a man and a woman. For example, when we say a husband and wife complement each other, we usually mean each has qualities that offset the weaknesses of the other. If one spouse is somewhat timid or bashful, the other may be more outgoing or gregarious. One's pensiveness may be offset by the other's spontaneity. Obviously, each partner is a complete human being, fully capable of independent living. But together, a new balance and new entity emerges.

In the area of medicine, however, things have historically been quite different. While attitudes are beginning to change, the prevailing interaction between scientific medicine and alternative medicine has not been congenial at all. Instead, too often each claims a monopoly on truth and healing, and each avoids the other at all costs.

Progress claimed by one camp is met with skepticism and rebuff by the other. These attitudes are fostered by ignorance and arrogance, since from the beginning each side has studiously avoided any dialogue with the other, and each feels it has the only valid approach.

Modern medicine is exemplified by the test tube, the sterile laboratory, the physician attired in a white lab coat, and the controlled clinical trial where various treatments are tested for efficacy. How could anyone have the audacity to suggest that any other approach could be of value? We apply our intellect, we design the appropriate scientific study, and then smart doctors coolly analyze the findings. The result is, supposedly, "objective truth," untainted by emotion or feeling. Surely this is how medicine should be done.

But the problem is that many of us, patients and physicians alike, have forgotten that scientific medicine has emerged as the standard of care only in this century. As a result, isn't it arrogant in the extreme to believe that prior to this "enlightened era," no real healing ever occurred?

If we are willing to concede that there are valid systems of health care that predate the scientific method, then it's worthwhile to understand their foundation. While scientific medicine is based upon the designed experiment and reproducibility of results, medicine of past centuries has a less concrete footing. Primitive healing systems are instead based upon feelings and experience. Observation is essential but not rigidly structured as in the scientific outlook. The ancient herbalist would prescribe remedies and consider the results. Over time, she would come to view certain prescriptions as useful in certain maladies and in certain types of patients. Healers shared their findings with one another. An oral tradition developed, and a sort of primitive pharmacopoeia emerged. There was no specific experiment that could be pointed to for verification; rather what occurred was the amassing of a commonly held body of wisdom. That truth, while not verified by rigid controlled studies, was validated instead by the collective experiences and feelings of the healers and their patients.

It's also important to note that healers in past centuries relied on a very personal relationship with the patient. In fact, I believe that much of the therapeutic effect of the treatment was inherently tied in with this trusting and caring relationship, and the essential underpinnings of that alliance were (and are) crucial to its effectiveness.

Conversely, Western medicine is based upon treatment modalities with specific effects—for example, the use of insulin in a patient with diabetes. A cascade of predictable and beneficial effects occur when insulin is given to a diabetic with an elevated blood sugar. The mindset of the patient or doctor is irrelevant in this setting. The effects of insulin are independent of either's expectations.

Alternative medicine is characterized by nonspecific effects. These are beneficial, ameliorating, and even healing. I do believe that many nonspecific effects are based upon the expectations or beliefs of those involved with using older treatments passed on through the ages—but this should not be minimized or discounted.

Much of the benefit of such medical systems is predicated upon the belief of the patient, the belief of the doctor, and the relationship between the two. The patient must expect that he is going to be helped, the caretaker must believe she will be helping the patient, and the two must have faith in each other. While the typical scientific physician would find such requirements foolhardy, many of us would consider the therapeutic effectiveness of such a scheme intuitively obvious.

While the herbalist would consider the physician-patient relationship crucial, the modern scientific physician may view it as of only marginal benefit. While the scientific physician prescribes specific agents for specific effects, the primitive healer, while having certain expectations, is more open to the unforeseen, the mysterious. While one system is based on hard facts, the other has a more empirical basis.

I think a new generation of healers is required. Whether one's training and approach are rooted in scientific or alternative medicine, a deep respect for and an understanding of the other's viewpoint will become mandatory. Even in China today, where both ancient and scientific philosophies exist side by side, there is pitifully little dialogue between the practitioners of the two disciplines. Despite proximity and a cultural tradition requiring that an educated person be both scientifically and artistically astute, China has two distinct medical systems with essentially no interaction.

The physician needs to see value in the ministrations of the herbalist and acupuncturist, who in turn must respect their more scientifically trained colleagues. Each must see the other as a caretaker. In short, pride in one's healing profession should not allow for disparagement of all others.

Doctors should view Western medicine as complete within the framework of the scientific approach which it employs. Similarly, the herbalist should view her system of healing as complete but again with the caveat that it too stems from a singular viewpoint. If human beings are indeed composed of the physical and spiritual, the mental and emotional, then no one perspective will encompass all truth.

An Overview of This Book

Rather than being presented in the typical dictionary-like format, the herbs in this book are discussed as groups, with each group sharing certain characteristics or similarities. In addition to delineating the particular qualities of a specific herb in the group, I also convey a general feeling about the group itself.

As a result, readers who wish to employ an herbal remedy will begin with the knowledge of which herbal group will be broadly applicable, and then may proceed to choose an herb with the specific subtleties required. The process is based therefore on knowledge and insight, as opposed to trial and error. This approach is far more rewarding and is much more likely to result in a favorable clinical effect.

The herbs considered in this book are useful for numerous common problems readers may face. By providing a general understanding of basic principles, and of herb groups and their characteristics, this book will also provide a strong framework to support an expanding knowledge in the area should you choose to pursue the subject further.

How to Read This Book

I believe it is important to read the entire book first. Then later you may go back to sections that particularly interest or concern you.

The book is divided into four parts. In Part One, I demonstrate the difference between the focuses of herbal medicine and modern scientific medicine. In herbal medicine, as we have seen, patients are considered largely responsible for the state of their own health and are viewed as multidimensional, comprising physical, mental, emotional, and spiritual realms. A logical corollary is that true health or wellness is achieved only when each level is vital and robust.

The human body is held in awe by herbalists. It is felt to have innate recuperative powers, and much of herbal therapeutics is directed at triggering these healing impulses. Similarly, normal bodily functions are respected, and everyday processes like eating, digestion, and elimination are used by the herbalist in an effort to maximize health. The goal is always to work with the body.

Herbal medicine also places great stock in the need for recuperation, which is far less emphasized in modern medicine, particularly with many managed care systems that rush people in and out of treatment. The problem is that energies are depleted not only by each encounter with disease but also by the pressures and demands of everyday living. Daily rest (something that is sometimes hard to get in our hectic culture!) is considered essential, and sufficient convalescence is mandatory after each occurrence of illness. In fact, a specific group of herbs (tonic herbs) is felt to have great revitalizing potential. They have no parallels or counterparts in Western medicine as generally practiced today.

Part Two groups together commonly used herbs for similar therapeutic medical problems. A basic understanding of the material in Part Two will greatly facilitate a rational choice of herbs for a host of common maladies.

In Part Three, I build on what has been discussed in the first two sections and present each of the major organ systems of the body, delineating the symptoms common to each and highlighting which herbals have been used effectively in each of these applications.

A key point to keep in mind is that while certain herbs have particular broad applications in disease states, subtle differences between herbs might make one or another more appropriate in individual cases. For example, while cramping pain in the digestive system generally responds favorably to drugs in the broad class of sedatives and antispasmodics, it is often found that chamomile is more effective for stomach cramping while hops are more effective when the intestine is involved. Thus in Part Three I utilize flowchart diagrams that always proceed from the more general symptom to the more specific.

In Part Four, we explore what is meant by a "complementary lifestyle." You are guided in the development of your own personal herbal prescription, a singular mixture to be used on a daily basis so that you can enjoy life to the fullest with maximal good health. We also review the basic tenets of herbal healing and their impact on everyday life, and my view that their widespread adoption would do much to promote wellness in our restless times.

Finally, we bring together herbal and scientific medicine to present a complementary approach to HIV disease and cancer.

PART *1*

In this section, I will present the herbal medicine approach to illness and contrast it with the Western perspective. As mentioned earlier, I firmly believe that both herbal medicine and Western medicine need to be considered together, rather than as mutually exclusive systems. Any system promulgating wellness that does not embrace both is inadequate.

The Herbal Mindset and Your Doctor: A Collaboration

*I*n this chapter, we'll discuss the overall mindset of the herbalist from ancient times to now, considering specific examples of illnesses and how they are regarded and treated by the herbalist. We'll also talk about working with your physician toward a complementary system of wellness—taking the best of both modern and ancient medicines.

The Herbal Mindset

Virtually all societies and cultures have used herbs for their medicinal properties. From before recorded time to the present and from the lush forests of South America to the arid deserts of the Middle East, plants have been esteemed for their curative effects.

It is undoubtedly true that each historic epoch and geographic locale develops its own distinctive worldview. Ancient Greek, Roman, and Chinese civilizations had different political systems, different moral or ethical norms, and different perceptions of our place in the cosmos. There were and are, however, certain common perceptions which emerged in primitive societies and ancient cultures regarding health and illness. While not identical, an overall commonality of approach justifies the use of the term "herbal mindset."

The underlying premise in a scientific worldview is that only the physical world counts. That means that if it can't be seen, heard, touched, or measured, a concept is of no consequence. We can employ the most sophisticated technology available, we can expand our vision at either extreme with the most expensive microscopes and telescopes, but in the end, if we can't see it, it doesn't matter.

According to the scientific model, then, illness is viewed in strictly physical terms. Pneumonia results when viruses or bacteria infect the lung; blockage of an artery supplying blood to the heart results in a heart attack. The therapeutic approach dictated by such a viewpoint is quite straightforward: an antibiotic to kill the bacteria or a surgical bypass around the blockage.

The attraction to the utility of such a model is immediately apparent. With concentrated study, cause and effect relationships can be discerned. Dedication and diligent research will ultimately result in appropriate interventions, and cures will be found. In this view, humans are physical beings, their afflictions are physical in nature, and their remedies will be accomplished by physical means. It's impossible to overstate the grand successes of this approach. Its achievements (penicillin, immunizations, surgeries) have benefited us all.

In societies where herbalism had its inception, humans were and are perceived in a different light. The physical nature of people cannot be denied; they are made of bone and muscle; they eat, breathe, and sleep. But they also have minds capable of thought and wonder, and they are subject to the gamut of emotions from melancholy to elation. From prehistory, humankind has surmised the existence of a spiritual realm and attempted to define its place and meaning in the cosmos. Traditionally, then, people are seen as a composite of physical, mental, emotional, and spiritual selves. For societies that emphasize alternative treatments, these multiple elements of the self are not seen as distinct and separate entities but rather as elements of a whole. Health requires vitality in all spheres, and infirmity results from disorder at any level. In many developing societies, physical illness is attributed to the malevolence of evil spirits. Disease is seen as affecting the entire being and at all levels: illness thus encompasses physical, mental, emotional, and spiritual realms.

This outlook has disadvantages. For example, it is much more complicated than the single-faceted scientific approach. While Western medicine has only to contend with the physical realm, alternative medicine deals with several others as well. Why, then, does herbalism survive and flourish today? And why are increasing numbers of Americans and Canadians, both patients and doctors alike, adopting the herbal mindset?

I believe that for many, such a perspective seems to explain things better or more precisely, and better portrays herbal supporters' view of reality. The scientific viewpoint is increasingly seen as incomplete. Let's look at a case of pneumonia. Two healthy young adults can be exposed to an organism that causes this infection, yet only one may become ill. Why? The explanation for this common occurrence depends on the particular viewpoint taken. The scientific physician will say that the patient who became ill was exposed to a greater number of bacteria or had a weaker immune system to fight off infection. Conversely, an herbal explanation could involve the mental outlook of the patient or his emotional state as having direct bearing on the clinical outcome; for example, let's say one person feels happy with his life while the other is extremely discontented and upset. The distressed person is generally more likely to become ill.

Here is another example. In my years as a practicing physician, I have treated hundreds of patients afflicted with cancer. I can unequivocally state that the patient's attitude toward her disease has a very direct bearing upon the outcome. Simply put, those patients who are confident and have a positive attitude do better than those who despair and have given up hope. Any honest physician will agree. Books have been written on the importance of an upbeat temperament (I particularly recommend *Anatomy of an Illness* by Norman Cousins). A five-part series presented on public television and entitled *Healing and the Mind* also received critical acclaim. It was hosted by Bill Moyers and is now available in book form. The whole area of mind-body medicine is receiving a great deal of attention today, including serious study by the National Institutes of Health.

Patient Outlook and Heart Attack

While scientifically verifiable risk factors (including elevated cholesterol level, high blood pressure, cigarette smoking, and diabetes) have received much attention, some physicians feel that these elements really don't explain why some people suffer heart attacks and others don't. These doctors feel that personality traits are critical in the development of heart disease. Thus, the aggressive, time-pressured, type A individual is much more likely to be affected than his more serene and placid neighbor.

Recently reported studies have confirmed that heart attacks are more likely to occur in the morning and most specifically on Monday mornings, and this is really not that surprising. Why? Because Monday morning is often the single most stressful time for working individuals. Association between the occurrence of illness and a period of increased pressure is very understandable to those with the herbal mindset.

Herbalism and Ancient Religion

Historically the practice of medicine was intimately related to religion and philosophy. In Asia, the Nei Ching, the ancient basic text of internal medicine, is also considered a source of great spiritual insight and is an important Taoist text.

In the Americas, herbalism has long been associated with ritual, magic, and the spiritual realm. Shamans are unique practitioners who are as much priests as healers. Entering into a trancelike or dream state by the use of psychoactive plants, they believed they were able to seek out the soul of the sick person and intuitively determine an appropriate therapy.

One cannot imagine an approach more removed from that of modern medicine. Consider an office visit with your primary care physician and contrast this with the drums, rattles, and incantations that form the basis of the shaman's craft. Yet, despite the incongruity of the scenes, some physicians today believe that prayer can definitely affect the course of disease.

One recent study divided patients who had a heart attack into two groups: one group was prayed for, the other was not. Patients were not told of their group assignment. The prayed-for group had fewer side effects than the group not prayed for. This is an area of active current research; many other studies have confirmed the positive effects of prayer. An exhaustive and fascinating summary of studies in this intriguing area can be found in the book *Healing Words* by Larry Dossey, M.D.

In short, the herbal mindset is holistic. It views illness and wellness from the perspective of intricate interactions of all the components that make up the complex person you call "me." It insists that people are a harmonious synthesis of the physical, spiritual, mental, and emotional elements and that each element must be given its due. Ignoring any one is a risk, sometimes a very serious one.

More than just "a strong mind in a strong body," this viewpoint insists that both emotional health and spiritual vigor are essential to maximum vitality. Self-esteem, the ability to forge and maintain trusting relationships, the capacity to love and be loved, and a sense of peace in the quietest of moments and in the deepest recesses of the soul are accordingly esteemed as major determinants of health.

Balance Is Important to Herbalists

Basic to the herbal mindset is the notion of balance. Wellness in alternative systems requires balance at many levels. In Ayurveda, the medicine of India, the vocation of the healer is to balance the three humors (fluids). This is accomplished, in part, by the judicious use of herbs and the prescription of appropriate diets. In Chinese medicine, illness is seen to result from an imbalance of yin and yang. Many Chinese physicians seek to manipulate these, largely through the use of herbs and acupuncture. In both systems, the balance of opposing forces results in maximal health and vigor. Greek medical tradition similarly sought to balance four bodily fluids and four temperaments. Hippocrates categorized herbs into four groups (hot, cold, damp, and dry) and taught that good health resulted in keeping these in balance.

Looking at our own lifestyles today, people need moderation and symmetry—just as they did a thousand years ago. No single aspect of human existence can be disregarded. Work must be balanced by play, exercise by rest, meditation by folly, and tears by laughter. All are integral to the human experience, and we must appreciate them all to be whole and healthy. The inherent wisdom of such an approach is being reaffirmed today.

On the physical level, we are beginning to appreciate the importance of exercise in preventing disease and extending vitality into the eighth and ninth decades of life. Similarly extolled are the benefits of moderating our intake of fats and sugars and the value of a diet emphasizing variety, especially of fruits and vegetables.

At a deeper and less intuitive level, similar lessons emerge. Balance is required in the mental realm as well, and the full range of human emotions are afforded significance. Ancient societies have always, for example, seen death as part of the cycle of life. Grieving was considered a natural process and sorrow an appropriate response to certain life situations. These were dealt with communally and were considered an essential if unpleasant part of mortal existence. The process of mourning was often ritualized and always respected. When completed, everyone was free to go on with life as before, surely with memories and recollections of the deceased but, because of a shared communal grieving, liberated from crippling and immobilizing ties to the departed.

But in our "feel-good" society, we often try to avoid the necessary process of bereavement and mourning. We do not allow ourselves to bring to consciousness our deepest emotions. We refuse to allow ourselves to let go and fully experience our pain and sorrow. Yet this is precisely what we must do in order to go on with the business of living and good health. Moments of sadness are an inherent part of mortal existence. Each of us will experience them; they are an inescapable aspect of the human condition. Rather than allowing life's sorrows to evoke denial and anger, we should approach them with acquiescence and consent. As it says in the book of Ecclesiastes, "For everything there is a season."

As any artist knows, light must be complemented by dark. As any composer knows, intensity and mood must vary to create beautiful music. In the wisdom of the ancients, happiness is incomplete and cannot be totally realized without sadness. To be human is to experience both fully in their time. Balance must be respected; mental health requires it.

I believe that the concept of balance is imperative as a broadly applicable principle, one validated by a variety of perspectives. Achieving balance is the major goal in all traditional systems of health and healing. Like all true wisdom, it is applicable in all places and at all times.

Using the Restorative Powers of Your Own Body

Another aspect of herbal thinking that differs from scientific methods of healing is the respect afforded the body's own restorative powers. For example, if you asked an M.D. how penicillin works, he would probably reply that it inhibits certain essential biochemical reactions in bacteria, causing their death and thus curing the infection.

An herbalist, in contrast, would more likely describe his ministrations as aiding the body in its own healing process. The human body has inherent curative properties and needs only to be encouraged in the proper direction. (Similarly, acupuncture is believed to balance or stimulate energy that is already innately present within the body.) This viewpoint is an essential component of the herbal mindset. Along with it is the corollary notion that a period of sickness depletes the body of much of its vitality and much of its healing potential. Thus a suitable period of recuperation, allowing the body to achieve its pre-illness state of vigor, is required after each encounter with disease.

I believe that modern medicine, which tends to attribute cure solely to its powerful drugs, dangerously underestimates the toll that illness actually takes on the human body. The battlefield of disease is the human organism itself, and the cure is often achieved via heroic physical bodily effort. Replenishment and renewal are necessary. I think lack of necessary recuperation encourages the epidemic of recurrent and chronic diseases rampant today.

It Is Important to Believe that Herbs Work

Belief in the herbal system seems to increase the efficacy of herbal treatments. Conceptually, I tend to view this as a logical consequence of several of the considerations discussed above. If you are open to the possibility of mind-body interaction, and if you can deal with the inherently inscrutable nature of many herbal effects, then in many cases your belief will increase the effectiveness of the herbal approach.

When two people are given a difficult chore to accomplish and one is convinced she can accomplish it while the other feels overwhelmed, we can predict who will succeed. A positive viewpoint is a major determinant of success. Similarly, the faithful believer will have an entirely different response to a religious service than the nonbeliever. Again, one's preconceptions have a profound effect on the experience.

The influence of belief on herbal effectiveness is best understood in the context of proposed herbal actions. Scientifically developed medications generally have a direct effect on bodily processes. They don't require our belief in them; their action is independent of our will.

Botanicals probably work primarily by encouraging and promoting natural healing processes. They help the body help itself. To be effective, then, they require at a minimum that the person wants to get better and that she also believes that herbs will help her in this effort. Only then will the inner capacity to heal be augmented and the body's recuperative imperative maximized.

Herbalism and Your Physician

To achieve a good complementary balance between modern medicine and herbalism, you need a cooperative physician, and increasing numbers of doctors are realizing the benefits of herbal therapy.

I have treated patients with a combination of modern medicine and herbs. For example, Marilyn (not her real name), age forty-one, had a serious problem with both tension headaches and arthritis. She was on a variety of medications prescribed by another doctor as well as up to twenty aspirins a day. And yet Marilyn felt that she wasn't making progress.

I started Marilyn on valerian for her headaches and fish oil capsules for her arthritis, and within a month, she described her response as "amazing." Marilyn was able to stop taking the prescription medications. She also slashed her aspirin consumption. She continues to take the valerian and the fish oil capsules.

In another case, Joyce, age forty-two, complained of very irregular periods and of severe swelling prior to the onset of her periods. She was very interested in being placed on a herbal regimen. I put Joyce on dong quai and uva ursi. Her periods became much more normal and her ankle swelling diminished considerably. Joyce has continued this regimen.

A dramatic case was the one of Mary, age seventy-eight. She had been on a variety of anti-inflammatory medications for her arthritis and felt little relief. On December 1, 1994, I put Mary on capsicum burdock and devil's claw, three times a day. Mary came back on December 15 and said she had already noted definite improvement. A satisfied herb user, Mary has continued with this regimen.

Obviously your doctor should not be expected to give up on modern medicine; for example, Marilyn still needed some aspirin for relief. And if I believed that Joyce or Mary would benefit from one of the modern treatments available today, I would have urged them to pursue that course in addition to the herbal treatments that have worked so well for all three women.

What if My Doctor Thinks Herbalism Is Weird?
Or I'm Afraid He Will?

Many people who would like to try herbal treatments are afraid that they could be harmful and never proceed, while others do take herbs but don't tell the doctor. The second course of action is the worse choice, because your physician needs to know what herbs you are taking to make sure they don't hide medical conditions for which you need treatment.

I strongly recommend that you do discuss herbal treatments with your primary care physician ahead of time. Do keep in mind, however, that doctors are human, and it's a good idea to realize that you could offend the doctor by rattling off how you're going to cure yourself. Medicine is, after all, your doctor's field.

Here's an approach that should work well with most doctors. When you see your doctor, tell her that you know that she has the medical degree, and not you. Be emphatic on this point. Obviously, she knows this is true, but it's important to convey the fact that *you* know it's true. Then tell her that you've been reading up on herbs and you'd really like to try whatever herb you are considering. Tell her you have seen some articles indicating that this herb may help a person with the illness from which you are seeking relief. When possible, show the doctor a bottle of the herb.

Now observe the reaction of your doctor. If you have been calm and respectful, in many cases your doctor will give you a cautious go-ahead. Or she may tell you that she'd like to research this herb further and get back to you. (That is actually a very positive response because now your doctor will be learning about herbs and can become a better partner in your health.)

In the worst case, your doctor may tell you that herbalism is trendy or bad and try to talk you out of it. If the doctor has a medical reason—for example, the herb you've selected would be harmful to you for a reason she can cite—then heed her opinion. However, if the primary objection appears to be bias and ignorance, and the doctor is extremely opposed to the use of any herbs for any reason, then you must make a difficult choice: whether to remain with this doctor and forgo the herbs or to find another physician who is more in tune with what you want as well as what you need.

In today's society, we can't depend on one doctor for life, and thus changes are sometimes necessary. You may find another physician who is willing to work with you on trying herbs, or, best case, a doctor who is knowledgeable about herbs and supports you in using them.

Your Herbalist May Not Like Doctors

If your information on herbs has come from someone who is not a medical doctor—perhaps someone with expertise in nutrition, chiropractic or some other field—you may find that the importance of modern medicine may be downplayed. Some herbalists believe that herbs and a positive mental attitude can cure anything.

Don't believe this. We still need modern medicine for all major ailments, such as cancer, heart disease, and a very broad array of illnesses too lengthy to list here. If your herbalist tells you that you don't need a physician but your common sense and your body tell you that you do, then go see your physician or at least call. Remember, the smart consumer doesn't depend solely on either ancient medicine or modern medicine, but instead relies on a complementary system, taking the best of each to achieve optimal health.

CHAPTER 2

Herbal Wellness versus Modern Medicine

*A*lternative medicine encourages self-reliance and maintaining good health—but it is inevitable that sometimes you will need to see your doctor. With effective use of botanicals, vitamins, and exercise, the time span between those visits to your doctor will probably be lengthened, which is good. But don't rely on herbs or other treatments to cure you of cancer or other serious illnesses. Herbs may be able to ease some of the symptoms of serious disease, but if surgery is the cure, then go to a surgeon. This is another example of complementary medicine, using the best of herbalism and modern medicine. Use common sense. For example, if you feel very ill, have a fever, and can't perform your normal tasks, you'd better see your physician.

We have all been advised of the folly of self-treatment. The adage "The physician who treats himself has a fool for a patient" applies to all, physician and layman alike. Yet the vast majority of diseases are self-limited, and if you are able to differentiate minor complaints from more serious conditions, encouragement of your body's own healing imperative may be all that is required.

Two major misconceptions plague the current Western approach to health care. First, we are too often reliant on the physician to heal every twinge of pain. Second, we feel that what we do between visits is largely irrelevant; if worse comes to worst and we again become sick, the physician will always be available for a cure. This is characteristic of the Western mindset. We go along, living from day to day paying little attention to our physical well-being. We become ill, see a physician, take her advice, get well, and once again become oblivious to matters of health. The consequences of what we do between doctors' appointments are, regretfully, ignored. In alternative medicine, however, one's lifestyle is given center stage.

In China there is a strongly held belief that both lifestyle and attitude significantly affect well-being. One's health in many ways depends on one's behavior and thought. In other words, health is a reflection of one's total lifestyle. Good health is the reward of leading a balanced life. Temperance in eating and drinking, moderate exercise, and spiritual and emotional harmony are perceived as the keys to longevity. Just as important as the specifics, however, is the notion inherent in all of the above: each of us is individually responsible for our own health.

A parallel viewpoint is seen in the Ayurvedic tradition, which developed in India. How you live, including your eating habits, work, social life, and even sexual activities are perceived as major determinants of health. The ancient Greeks also believed that maintenance of good health required a balanced diet and that daily exercise and fresh air were essential to maximum vitality. Early Roman medicine, highly influenced by the Greeks, espoused similar notions. The common thread is the important role we each play in maintaining our own good health.

Today similar ideas are being voiced in the Western world and fortunately finding a receptive audience. For example, we all know that smoking is tantamount to slow suicide, regular exercise is beneficial, and a high-fat diet promotes many of the ills that plague us. Translating this knowledge into lifestyle changes can be a demanding process, but people are starting to pay attention. Similarly, most of us intuitively know that emotional equilibrium and spiritual serenity contribute positively to good health. Today's strong interest in mind-body medicine reveals that a sensitive chord has been struck and people are beginning to realize that a positive mental state beneficially affects the healing process.

It's not necessarily easy to attain a positive mental attitude; this may require a concerted effort. But the proliferation of peer groups, support groups, self-help groups, and the like attest to our belief in the need for emotional equanimity and its role in possible recovery. Health is the result of sensible, ordered, disciplined living, day in and day out. All realms of being—physical, mental, emotional, and spiritual—are involved. The burden of health is lifted off the healer's shoulders and borne happily by the patient. Happily, since with the added responsibility also comes the opportunity to be the architect of one's well-being.

We have all experienced sickness. Likewise we can all recall days when we felt full of life and vitality, when we were at our peak physically and mentally. Most of our time, however, is spent somewhere in the middle. There is an easily recognized continuum from maximum vitality to terminal illness. But keep in mind that the absence of sickness is not at all the same as being healthy. Health in this sense implies a feeling of *maximum wellness*. Herbalists insist that people who live a balanced life cannot help but feel most alive and vibrant. Those whose lives are a balance of work and play, exercise and rest, who are temperate in all their appetites, who are at peace emotionally and spiritually will enjoy long and healthy lives.

All this makes good sense. However, in emphasis it is radically opposed to typical Western ideas. The basic tenet of modern medicine is that disease is the result of an external agent, something separate and apart from ourselves. The emphasis, then, is on the other, and we are acted upon rather than masters of our fate. But for herbalists, the emphasis is on the self—an imbalance or disorder in one's whole life pattern that predisposes to disease. These are radically different starting points when dealing with issues of health and disease.

Not surprisingly, the two approaches have also given rise to entirely different therapeutic approaches. For example, because modern medicine perceives the disease as an external entity, it is treated as an enemy. Thus the disease and its symptoms are surgerized, cauterized, irradiated, and medicated in a full frontal attack to get rid of the enemy, and the bulk of the effort goes into fighting the disease. Herbalists approach the problem from an entirely different perspective. The emphasis is on the person; the body and its basic functions are respected. Certain symptoms (for example, fever, cough, vomiting, and diarrhea) are seen as *positive attempts* the body is making to thwart a disease. These are not, therefore, suppressed unless causing a person considerable discomfort. But modern medicine struggles to get rid of your cough, diarrhea, fever, and so forth. Most modern physicians want to rid you of the symptoms of the illness as well as the illness itself.

This is ironic since modern medicine has also affirmed that many of the body's defenses work at maximum efficiency at an approximate temperature of 101 degrees. As a result, suppressing a modest fever may also repress your natural immune mechanism that is geared to ridding the body of infection. (Please note: High fever can be dangerous, and a physician should always be consulted in such cases.)

Some physicians do realize that it's important to allow the symptoms of the illness to occur. For example, most lung specialists generally encourage the cough reflex in cases of pneumonia. They are thus supporting the body's urge to rid itself of infecting bacteria.

A more dramatic illustration may provide further insight. A patient is brought to the emergency room following multiple stab wounds. He has lost a great deal of blood, has no obtainable blood pressure, and is in shock. For the past thirty years, a well-rehearsed script would be played out in this clinical setting: placement of a large intravenous line and replacement of the fluids that have been lost due to hemorrhage. The accepted dogma is that one must immediately put back what has been lost, restore the patient's blood pressure so that organ function can be maintained, and take the victim to surgery.

But a report published in the *New England Journal of Medicine* in October 1994 boldly challenged the accepted doctrine. This report divided trauma patients into two groups. In one group, the above protocol of rapid fluid replacement was followed. In the second group, no fluids were administered prior to surgery.

Only a physician who has spent time in an emergency room caring for such patients could appreciate how radical a departure from accepted therapy this is. Aggressive intravenous replacement in trauma patients with blood loss and low blood pressure represents hallowed medical tradition.

So what did the study reveal? The validated, statistically verified results showed that fluid replacement was detrimental and that the patients receiving aggressive intravenous therapy had more complications and a higher death rate.

Why? Without treatment, as blood loss progresses, blood pressure drops and the velocity of blood flow diminishes. This affords maximal opportunity for the body's clotting mechanism to come into play. A thrombus (blood clot) forms at the site of bleeding and further hemorrhage is thus stopped. The body has effectively stabilized a potentially lethal situation. Rapid fluid replacement, on the other hand, could either prevent thrombus formation (by diluting clotting factors or increasing blood flow) or (by an increase in pressure) mechanically disrupt a thrombus already formed. The body unerringly initiates life-saving mechanisms on its own, and this study indicates that, at times, aggressive human intervention is counterproductive.

My point is not to malign science. Certainly surgical intervention is required in all cases of trauma. Additionally, good sense has dictated what has been standard medical therapy over the last thirty years. However, as we gain in understanding of more subtle physiological mechanisms, we may develop a more profound respect for the body's innate healing capacity and be less inclined to interfere at every possible opportunity.

A fundamental belief of herbal medicine is that the body should not be prohibited from its own curative efforts. It sees much of today's chronic disease as a result of unresolved battles where suppression of uncomfortable symptoms by palliative medications has prevented the elimination of the disease by the body's natural defenses. If the body is believed to possess self-correcting principles, then the function of natural herbs must be to encourage these processes.

In the scientific model, you are a static recipient, prey to foreign influences that can cause disease, and subjected to a variety of invasive procedures. In the herbal model, you are an active participant in your own health, which in most cases is largely determined by your own lifestyle and attitude.

When you become ill, you will respect your body's attempts at healing. And you will recognize that you, more than anyone or anything, will determine the outcome. The potential of this approach is only now being rediscovered.

Herbal Medications
versus Modern Drugs

A basic respect and even an awe for the human body is at the root of herbal treatment. The body is believed to have innate recuperative healing properties that herbs are felt to stimulate. In herbalism, there is a basic and implied faith that the body's natural response will effect a cure more surely than human interventions.

In most Western religions a contrasting notion is widely accepted. The prevalent perception is that, as a result of the sins of humankind, the body is prey to suffering and disease and is considered debased and stripped of its full potential. This perspective makes reliance on the body difficult.

If human nature is seen in the great Western religious traditions as corrupted by the sins of our forebears, then dependence on the body's inherent healing tendencies appears irrational. The body is viewed as an unclean vessel, the insatiable source of temptation and sin, the major obstacle to our finding true serenity. It can hardly be relied upon to ease our pain or effect a cure.

Additionally, the prevalent Western philosophical perspective sees humanity composed of a separate mind and body. In this scheme the mind is afforded supremacy. Thus, reliance on study, learning, research, and science will provide the antidote to disease and death. Such a view encourages acceptance of the Western model of health and disease. Dependence on the body to cure itself is folly.

Accordingly, the religious and philosophical underpinnings of Western sensibility discourage any great dependence on the body as a source of wellness or cure. I'm not suggesting that we are consciously thinking about such things when we are ill. Rather, they represent part of a prevailing worldview that is an ingrained and integral part of our subconscious notions about the human condition.

Herbalists believe that the body holds inherent self-correcting tendencies to heal. Herbs are perceived as acting in synergy with the body to effect improvement or even cure. Keep in mind that throughout the world even today, the majority of medicines taken are herbal remedies.

Many herbs have been used for thousands of years. Compare that to today's pharmaceuticals. Every few years there is a new batch of antibiotics, antiarthritic drugs, heart medications, antiulcer drugs, and so on, which largely replace those that preceded them.

A physician who practiced only twenty or thirty years ago would be baffled by the vast majority of medicines in use today. In stark contrast, many of the herbs used today are the same as those used by Hipppocrates and Galen two or three thousand years ago. A common expression used to denote quality is "It stood the test of time." Herbal therapeutics most certainly has done that.

Alternative methods of treatment have developed independently all over the world. Herbal practice formed the basis not only of Asian medicine but also of Greek, Roman, Islamic, European, and North and South American Indian healing. In addition to what we know of recorded history, there is also anthropological evidence of herb usage in the earliest, most primitive communities.

In short, the use of herbs has been universal both geographically (throughout the world), and temporally (from the beginning of history to the present time). It is easy, however, to understand how prescription medications have assumed a dominant role in the West.

First, there was the discovery of antibiotics to cure formerly lethal infectious diseases. Then came the use of vitamins to cure disabling and sometimes fatal deficiency syndromes, followed by a multitude of other powerful tools added to the physician's arsenal.

There was something neat, clean, and precise about these new medicines. In comparison, plant remedies seemed crude and lacked the cool efficiency of drugs. Drugs created by pharmaceutical companies fit better with our new scientific outlook at the turn of the century.

But our viewpoint has changed, and many of us no longer view science so beneficently. Perhaps our current disillusionment with modern medicine is part of a broader current discontent with science as a whole. We have now had time to learn that science has a downside. For example, bacteria can develop resistance to antibiotics and newer, stronger ones must be created, which can have powerful side effects. In addition, the latest modern medications can be very expensive.

Perhaps the current interest in herbal medicine represents an urge to return to a simpler time. It may even be that the prevailing worldview in the West is beginning to change. Mind and body are considered less as distinct entities than as different aspects of the same self. We are beginning to see ourselves less in national terms and more as members of the same human community. We are beginning to define our relationship to our environment as caretakers rather than plunderers. Underlying much of this fresh outlook is a new respect for things we have all too often taken for granted. A new respect for the body is engendering a greater appreciation of its full potential and the desire to make the most of it.

I am not suggesting that modern medicine be abandoned. I do believe that it is consulted too frequently, called upon unnecessarily, and relied on far too often when all that is needed is a little faith in the body's recuperative powers and a little encouragement of them. Perhaps faster and stronger medicine is not always best.

Categorizing Herbs

Although we will be categorizing herbs and putting them into various groups, divisions must be seen as somewhat arbitrary. Two important aspects of herbal remedies must be kept in mind. First, all herbs have a multitude of effects. Angelica, for example, is most often used for its gastrointestinal effects and is usually classified as a digestive. However, it is also a warming drug (diaphoretic) and has expectorant properties (aids in the clearing of the lungs) and could just as well be listed in those groups.

In all cases, I will try to list herbs with respect to their major or most useful effects, remembering that they also may have other beneficial properties. In addition to having a multitude of effects, the overall merit and efficacy of an herb is greater than the sum of its parts, and this is a second important precept of herbal therapy.

Herbal Effects on Bodily Functions

*T*his chapter will deal with the basic life processes affected by herbs and will describe how herbs become part of an overall healing strategy. The simplicity and common sense of the herbal approach will become quite apparent. I will concentrate on the four areas that represent the foundation of much of herbal therapy: vitality and energy, elimination, temperature, and restoration. Most mixtures or formulas contain herbs that affect one or more of these areas.

Vitality and Energy

The concept of vital energy is basic to all forms of non-Western practices, including herbal treatments and acupuncture. It has various names in different cultures but in all cases the idea is the same. The vital energy differentiates life from death. In China it is called *qi* (pronounced "chi"). Those who have a balanced *qi* possess a strong positive vitality. In Western terms, we would say they are resistant to disease.

Qi comes in three basic denominations: original *qi* (transmitted from your parents), nutritional *qi*, and air *qi*. Original *qi* is obtained only once, but nutritional *qi* and air *qi* are used and replenished daily.

Qi *and Digestion*

The gastrointestinal system (gut) has always been a major focus of herbal remedies. It is here that digestion and absorption take place. It is here that nutritional energy is restored and vital energy is renewed. Any system of healing that relies on the body's natural activities must also ensure an adequate store of vitality and energy to fuel these processes. You need to have sufficient nutritional *qi* to overcome disease or illness.

As a result, herbal prescriptions often begin with plants having a major effect on digestive processes. Two classes of herbs dramatically influence digestion and absorption: the aromatic digestives and the bitter digestives. These will be discussed at length in later chapters, along with the rationale for favoring one group over the other. It is sufficient for now to say that virtually any herbal mixture lacking a digestive stimulant is incomplete.

Herbs that increase circulation, such as the peripheral vasodilators and circulatory stimulants, aid in the delivery of vital energy and nutrients throughout the body as they contribute to vitality. They are part of any herbal prescription when coldness or impaired circulation is a problem.

It must be noted here that the concept of vital energy in ancient cultures extends beyond the physical. Vital energy in traditional societies is believed to encompass and be supported by friendship, art, beauty, love, and spirituality. All of these are considered essential to good health; shortcomings in one or more of these areas are believed to lead to illness.

Elimination

Removal, or excretion of waste materials, is central to herbal practice, and many herbal formulas will promote elimination. Why? Because we are awash in a sea of toxins, both internally generated (waste material) and in the external environment (food additives, pollutants, radiation, and so on). Modern medicine can attest to the disease-producing potential of these chemicals. Two examples will illustrate the effects of these toxins. Diabetic coma is the result of an excessive accumulation of acids generated by the body; lead poisoning results from an excessive exposure to lead in the environment.

Herbalists see accumulations of toxins as commonplace in disease states, so they seek to augment the body's natural tendency to eliminate these poisons. A basic tenet of herbal medicine may be stated quite succinctly: "better out than in." Thus elimination processes are encouraged.

In the past, some efforts at elimination were quite dramatic. American Indians constructed sweat lodges in order to induce a fever and profuse sweating. Powerful emetics were given to induce vomiting, and strong laxatives and enemas were employed as cleansing agents.

While such vigorous attempts at elimination have been largely excluded from contemporary herbalism, and an herbal mixture may not contain a specific herb for elimination, most herbal mixtures do encourage a mild cleansing or discharge of toxins. Remember that herbs have multiple effects. Many plants have constituents that are excreted in the urine and act as diuretics. They induce a flow of urine and aid in the elimination of toxins via this route.

Other plants act as diaphoretics and provoke a mild sweat, carrying harmful material out of the body. In addition, mild laxatives may be used when normal eliminative function seems to be impaired. Cholagogues, which stimulate the secretion of bile, are believed to be particularly useful in the treatment of liver disease. Cough is encouraged and supported by the use of expectorants. It is not suppressed.

Temperature

No consideration of herbal therapeutics could ignore a discussion of "hot" and "cold" because these are among the most basic primitive concepts regarding health and disease. From earliest times, heat was associated with life (the sun) and cold was associated with disease or death (a corpse is cold).

Herbalists regard fever as a normal healthy bodily response, perceiving that the fevered body is actively engaged in a battle against disease. As a result, herbalists support fever and don't seek to suppress it. Instead, the goal is to maintain the body at optimal fever temperature (101–102 degrees). If the patient's temperature goes above 101–102 degrees, it can be brought down by using cooling remedies like bitters or by employing a tepid bath.

In addition to body temperature, we also consider an illness to be either hot or cold depending on the patient's basic response. A cold illness is one characterized by a subdued bodily response. It is marked by fatigue, lassitude, underactive metabolism and sluggishness. It will require warming herbs (vasodilators or aromatic digestives). Conversely, a hot illness is characterized by excessive response. It is marked by anxiety, nervousness, excessive energy, and an overactive metabolism and will require cooling herbs (bitter digestives, sedatives, and antispasmodics).

Many herbalists feel that to be successful, an herbal remedy must contain a constituent that will counteract the basic temperature of the illness. A practical application of the notion of hot and cold in the formulation of an herbal prescription is presented in a simple and straightforward manner in Chapters 6 and 32.

Restoration

The herbalist believes that every encounter with disease takes something out of the patient, depleting vital energy that consequently must be restored. In ancient medicine, a period of recuperation was generally applied to all patients after any condition. Neglect of this basic premise is probably one of the major shortcomings and most serious errors of modern medicine today because most modern physicians fail to take into account the toll that an illness has taken on the patient.

In fact, I believe that failing to consider the need for the body to recuperate contributes to the myriad of chronic conditions that plague us today. We remain weakened after an illness and are then unable to mount an adequate defense in our subsequent encounters with disease. Thus an acute illness that should be easily overcome becomes a lingering chronic problem. Chronic hepatitis, chronic Epstein-Barr virus, chronic fatigue syndrome, and chronic respiratory or gastrointestinal problems barely represent the tip of the iceberg.

The vast majority of office visits to all health care practitioners are for chronic conditions. If we allowed ourselves adequate recuperation after each illness and worked at restoring our own vital energy to pre-illness levels, I believe that the modern scourge of chronic debilitating disease could be largely eliminated.

The following recuperative principles can be applied at all times and need not be limited to periods of convalescence.

Rest is the cornerstone and most important revitalizing principle. Often a short period of rest is all that is needed to begin to reverse a chronic condition. After any acute illness, a few days' rest is imperative, and more protracted illnesses will require a more prolonged convalescence. Be attuned to your body. It will tell you when you need rest and when you are ready to resume. You need only listen.

Exercise, somewhat paradoxically, is also essential to a successful restorative regimen. Periods of exercise will improve the quality of rest and prevent a buildup of excess nervous energy and anxiety. It will also provide for the balance which is so necessary in all aspects of life: rest needs to be offset with exercise. If your condition is extremely debilitated, perhaps you can begin with a leisurely stroll. In most cases, ten to fifteen minutes of moderate exercise (such as walking) for one or more times daily should be initiated. When fully recovered, a regular routine of aerobic exercise for approximately 30 minutes 3 to 4 times a week should become a permanent part of your lifestyle.

Proper diet will also hasten recuperation. Certain foods have been ascribed restorative powers. These include raw fruits and vegetables (particularly in summer), fish, poultry, and yogurt. Hearty stews and soups are considered therapeutic in winter. Avoid fatty foods and refined carbohydrates. Fresh unadulterated foods should be chosen over those with preservatives and additives. Avoid caffeine and alcohol.

These recommendations need not be confined to periods of convalescence but can also be used as the basis for a lifetime of wellness.

Tonic herbs are believed to have restorative properties and to revitalize organs weakened by illness. In addition to their role in convalescence, these herbs are used daily by many as part of a program of preventive medicine to maintain a state of maximum well-being. These herbs will be discussed in detail later.

Summary

An herbal prescription will affect a variety of physiological processes to maximize the body's natural healing powers. Typically the herbal prescription will help to increase digestion and absorption of nutrients, aid in the elimination of toxic materials, and provoke a gentle heating or cooling as required by the illness being treated. This strategy forms the basis for most herbal prescriptions. Other herbs may be added for specific symptomatic effects, but everything is done naturally, in accordance with normal bodily processes. The goal in herbal medicine is simply to help the body help itself.

PART 2

This section begins with some practical suggestions on purchasing herbs. Don't be concerned with memorizing details, but rather work to acquire a feeling for the effects of the various groups presented.

CHAPTER 5

Buying Herbs

*I*n earlier times, how to use herbal remedies was largely a "do it yourself" endeavor. You would begin by first growing and then drying your own plants. These then require storage, usually in dark airtight bottles and in a cool dry place. Even under the best of circumstances, loss of potency occurs with time, and such herbs become largely ineffective after about a year. Even with well-prepared dried herbs, you are still faced with the task of extracting the active ingredients and preparing the herb in such a way that it could be taken easily and with a minimum of distaste.

Thus infusions, decoctions, extractions, and tinctures were arduously prepared by dedicated proponents of herbal therapy in the past. Purists today continue this tradition, and their dedication is to be applauded. You may one day decide to prepare your own remedies with similar zeal but, at least initially, I recommend more "user friendly" options.

With the increase in interest in herbal therapy, there has been a parallel growth in the availability of ready-to-use herbal products. Once relegated to health food stores and specialty shops, herbal medicines are now increasingly available in pharmacies and even some supermarkets. In this book I have specifically tried to concentrate on herbs that are widely available.

Herbs can be purchased in a variety of forms. Generally, the way the herb is processed and sold is less important than the integrity and quality of the herb manufacturer. Larger companies now sell standardized products with guaranteed potency. These are the herbs most widely available through pharmacies and food stores.

Owners of the smaller, more specialized shops may purchase from more modest suppliers, but they are extremely concerned about herbal quality since it is a major part of their business. Thus, if you rely on either the larger chain stores or the more specialized shops, you can be quite confident that you are getting quality products.

There are several advantages inherent to herb shops, however, that may even warrant going a little out of your way to find one. The first is that they will have a greater variety of herbs available. Frequently, the proprietors have very strong feelings about herbalism and are enthusiastic proponents of its benefits. Equally important, they are often very knowledgeable about herbs, anxious to share that information with you, and glad to answer any questions you may have. For an initiate into the herbal lifestyle, an hour spent in an herb shop can be most rewarding.

Teas

Of the varied forms in which herbs are available, teas may be the most familiar. Chamomile tea is readily available in almost all food stores, and many other herbs (including peppermint, hops, and fennel) are available in this form.

Teas are an ideal way to take herbs meant to relax or relieve anxiety. The simple act of making and enjoying a hot drink provides a break in the rush and turmoil of daily life, adding to the therapeutic effect. When you prepare the tea, do not use boiling water because this can cause loss of valuable volatile oils. Generally the tea is steeped for approximately ten minutes. While enjoying a relaxing herbal beverage, please remember that you are taking a medication, and don't exceed the recommended dosage. This is especially important for products bought in health food stores or herb shops, which tend to be more potent than those from the grocery. I would advise using herbal teas as needed, but don't exceed three or four cups per day.

Capsules or Tablets

Many of the more widely used herbs are available in capsules or tablets. These are convenient and easy to use, so new devotees often prefer to take herbs in these forms. Generally, instructions are given on the bottle, for example "Take 1 to 3 capsules, 1 to 3 times a day." Always follow label instructions, starting at the lower dosage range.

Extracts

Extracts are herbal preparations manufactured by soaking herbs in an alcohol solution. They are usually available in dropper bottles.

Typically you mix a number of drops with a small amount of water. As with capsules and tablets, a dosage range is usually given, and the same caveats apply.

A particular benefit of extracts is their ease of use in the formulation of herbal mixtures. You can combine the appropriate number of drops of each herb with a small amount of water and take them together. Making individualized herbal mixtures is greatly facilitated with this method, the one I personally prefer.

Powders

Some herbs are sold as powders. Stores that sell them in this form usually also carry empty capsules to facilitate administration. Alternatively, powders can be mixed with water or juice. Powders are generally less convenient than capsules and tablets, which will increasingly replace them in the future.

Dried Herbs

The dedicated herbalist can obtain dried herbs. These likewise can be put in capsules or brewed as a tea. Their major drawback, however, is storage. Generally they must be bought in bulk and, as mentioned previously, stored in airtight containers and kept out of direct sunlight. While powders and dried herbs are unquestionably effective, the novice herbalist is probably best served by the less daunting extracts, capsules, or teas.

Mixtures

Combination products (mixtures) are also available. In these, groups of herbs that benefit a given function (for example, the heart or immune system) are combined by the manufacturer into a single capsule (or tea bag).

As a careful reader of this book, you will be equipped to develop your own herbal formula specific to your particular needs and precisely fitting your temperament. One of the great rewards of reading this book will be your ability to formulate a personal herbal mixture to maximize your own well-being and help ensure your continued good health. This is covered in detail in Chapter 32.

Topical Herbs

Lastly, certain herbs can be applied directly to the skin and can be advantageously employed in a whole host of minor skin irritations. The most effective and widely available of the topical herbs are discussed in Chapter 18.

I have purposely chosen, in most cases, to omit doses in this book. Dosage of any herbal product varies according to the form used, preparation by the manufacturer, potency, and so on, so follow directions on the bottle. As with any form of herbal remedy, I advise starting at the lower end of recommended doses and increasing as needed and tolerated.

This chapter is not intended to be an exhaustive presentation of all the forms that herbal remedies can take. Such an approach could prove intimidating and needlessly delay your pursuit of natural remedies. Rather, I have tried to keep things simple while giving you more than enough information to walk into an herb shop, health food store, pharmacy, or supermarket and begin your quest for herbal wellness.

A Useful Herbal Classification

*W*e will now begin the material that will give you a basic understanding of herbs. In each of the following chapters, you will learn the primary actions of a basic herb group. Several herbs are presented in each group. While sharing properties common to the group, their individual nuances and subtleties will be highlighted. I believe that such a presentation will enable you to think about herbs in a useful and organized manner. Understanding the basic characteristics of the herb groups provides the information base you need to formulate sound, sensible, and effective herbal remedies.

Most herbs have a myriad of effects, and any grouping of herbs based on physiological actions is somewhat arbitrary. Some herbalists may argue with some (or even many) of the particulars in the following chapters, but the following classification seemed to me to be the most workable.

Again, the main value of this approach is that it provides a viewpoint or focus for looking at herbs in an organized manner and formulating a mixture based upon an understanding of herbal principles. This approach is far preferable to thumbing through a list of herbs and randomly selecting three or four because they sound appropriate—but with no understanding of their basic properties.

Herbal medicine has been practiced for thousands of years. Through a vast and colorful history it has been learned that certain herb groups work best when used with other specific groups, and that certain conditions should be treated with one group of herbs and not another despite some shared properties in the two groups.

I hope that this chapter and the next several chapters will make all this quite clear and that you will derive not only improved health but also a real sense of satisfaction from formulating your own herbal remedies based on sound herbal therapeutic principles. This is a serious endeavor requiring thought, sensitivity, and judgment, but by adhering to the basics being presented and listening to your own body, I think you will be quite gratified with the results.

As a physician, I have worked hard to encourage my patients to take responsibility for their own health. I have always felt that if I explain why I am asking a patient to do something (for example lose weight, stop smoking), then compliance improves.

In a very real sense, our own life span is often determined largely by what we eat and drink, and how we work and play. Lifestyle choices are often good predicters of the diseases that will ultimately do us in. I find myself spending more and more time discussing such choices with my patients and am always amazed to find that they are surprised by the information I give them. I find the whole area of patient education extremely enjoyable and, as I said, very worthwhile since it often favorably affects patient behavior.

I also want to educate you in the proper use of herbs. I am convinced that by carefully reading this short section you will gain a solid foundation of herbal knowledge and the confidence that goes along with it. You will be anxious to use herbs as part of a daily wellness prescription and be comfortable in calling on them in times of infirmity. We usually know little about our acquaintances but a good friend is someone we know well. Get to know the herbs well and they will become trusted friends.

The Herbal Groups

Aromatic digestives

Bitter digestives

Vasodilators

Sedatives and antispasmodics

Diuretics

Expectorants

Cleansing herbs

Tonic herbs

Chinese tonic herbs

Male hormonal herbs

Female hormonal herbs

Herbs used topically (on the skin)

Concepts of Hot and Cold

In addition to the more practical groupings just listed, one further grouping is of more nostalgic significance. It is based upon the ancient principles of "hot" and "cold," briefly mentioned in Chapter 4.

Galen, the ancient Greco-Roman physician, believed that the temperature of illnesses was of great importance, and he also categorized herbs according to their temperament. While his rigorous consideration is a valued piece of medical memorabilia, I consider this particular classification to be of mainly historical interest.

A hot illness was believed to be characterized by fever or a fiery, vigorous bodily response. Examples are the commonly encountered infectious diseases (for example influenza, strep throat, pneumonia, ear infections, and even the common cold). Acute illnesses (those of sudden onset and short duration) also tend to fall into the hot category. All these are believed to respond to treatment with cooling herbs.

In contrast, a cold illness was believed to evoke a blunted or underactive response. Chronic illnesses (for example, chronic fatigue syndrome or chronic hepatitis and debilitating diseases like cancer and AIDS) also are considered in the cold category. These need to be countered by warming herbs.

From my perspective, far more significant is your basic personality, your basic temperament. In general, the aggressive, anxious, excitable, agitated, nervous type (that is, most of us today) will benefit most from cooling herbs, while those fortunate few who are more placid or passive will respond best to warming herbs.

I mention the notions of hot and cold primarily for the sake of completeness. Aside from some practical suggestions on hot and cold herbs that are noted throughout this book, your choice of herbs will depend primarily on your symptoms and the herb effects that you require. By correctly choosing the herb that best treats your particular symptoms at a given time, you will almost automatically choose an herb whose temperature is appropriate.

The Warming Herbs

Aromatic digestives

Vasodilators

The Cooling Herbs

Bitter digestives

Sedatives and antispasmodics

A reasonable approach to an herbal remedy often begins with choosing an appropriate digestive aid. The goal here is to increase the absorption of nutrients, increase the vital energy (which will be needed to overcome the illness), and provide a soothing effect on the gut. Virtually any herbal mixture for use in health or illness is based on an appropriate digestive herb. Thus most herbal mixtures will begin with either a warming aromatic digestive or cooling bitter digestive.

Your symptoms may dictate the addition of either a vasodilator or an herb from the sedative and antispasmodic group. Typically, to round out an herbal mixture you would then add one or more herbs specifically geared to the symptoms present. For example, if cough is prominent, an expectorant would be added. Or if joint pain is prominent, a cleansing herb would be indicated.

The more specific components of a formula will be discussed as we go through each of the herbal groups in this section of the book. In addition, Part Three is a systematic presentation of herbs useful in treating the most commonly encountered symptoms and is arranged by the body's organ systems. Although these herbs can be used as singles (alone), their combination with other herbs and the formulation of an individualized mixture to suit the user's particular temperament is encouraged.

Don't be concerned if this all seems confusing at first. It will all become quite concrete and clear in Chapter 32, which provides a simple, step-by-step approach to formulating an herbal mixture. There you will learn how to prepare a personal herbal prescription for everyday use. It will be your wellness prescription to maximize your vitality and ability to enjoy life. By simply adding specific herbs for specific problems and perhaps deleting or substituting others, it can also act as the basis for mixtures to treat the occasional illnesses we all suffer.

The end result could not be more fulfilling; you will be helping your body to achieve its maximum wellness.

Aromatic Digestives

*7*he first group of herbs we will consider is the aromatic digestives. The aromatic digestives, as a group, all favorably influence the absorption and assimilation of food. They all increase
appetite and act favorably on digestion. Additionally they increase
secretions and encourage the normal forward movement of food in
the gut (peristalsis).

The end result is an increase in the availability of foodstuffs to
the body and an increase in vital energy. When you are ill, the main
benefit of aromatic digestives is their fortifying effect. They are also
useful when taken during convalescence, when the body is in a
weakened state. Then they act to revitalize the body, restoring it to
its state of former vigor.

One of the digestive herbs might reasonably form the basis of almost any herbal mixture. The choice between the aromatic digestives
and the bitter digestives will depend on the basic temperature of the
disease being treated. Since the aromatic digestives are warming in
nature and mildly stimulating, they are used whenever these effects
are desirable.

We will consider four herbs in this category: cardamom, cinnamon, angelica, and fennel, pointing out the unique qualities of each
that would lead to its use in specific conditions. Rather than just listing the effects of an herb, I will try to convey a feeling for its overall
quality or essence.

CARDAMOM

Cardamom is very useful as an aid to increase appetite. It has a definite warming effect but is only mildly stimulating. These properties,
along with its favorable actions on digestion and absorption, make
it an ideal herb for patients who are chronically ill, especially those
in whom poor appetite and digestion are particular problems.

In addition, cardamom has a reputation for being useful in

pregnancy, particularly for morning sickness and headache. Cardamom therefore is a useful aromatic digestive whose particular niche is for those who are more chronically disabled and for gastrointestinal problems related to pregnancy.

CINNAMON

Cinnamon, like cardamom, is useful in treating chronic conditions. It is particularly useful, however, in the treatment of uncomfortable gastrointestinal symptoms. It has a pronounced antigaseous effect, relieves abdominal pain secondary to spasm, and has antidiarrheal properties. Cinnamon was used by the Greeks, Romans, and Biblical Hebrews in the treatment of indigestion, and its medicinal qualities are noted in Chinese herbals dating back to 2700 B.C.

Like other herbs in this class, cinnamon not only is a digestive aid but also pacifies intestinal hyperactivity. These qualities, along with the fact that it is quite warming, make it an ideal herb for the very commonly encountered viral gastrointestinal problems characterized by chills, abdominal pain, colic, and diarrhea. It is also useful in other flulike conditions characterized by chills or feeling cold.

ANGELICA

Angelica has properties quite similar to those of both cardamom and cinnamon. It is useful in both acute and chronic conditions that are centered in the digestive system. Thus it can be used both in states of convalescence or in the treatment of acute gastrointestinal discomfort. In addition, angelica has considerable properties as an expectorant. It has a prominent action in drying up excessive lung secretions, and it aids in their expectoration.

As with all aromatic digestives, angelica is warming in nature, and when used in infections, it is believed to encourage a therapeutic sweat. Thus angelica is a most useful herb in dealing with viral infirmities of the digestive tract or lungs.

FENNEL

Fennel is most useful in calming intestinal cramps and excessive stomach gas. It has been used effectively for centuries in the treatment of colic in infants. It also effectively suppresses hiccups. Fennel is believed to be a useful appetite stimulant as well, and it may be used to help increase desire for food in the elderly. In addition, it is believed to have hormonal effects and to encourage breast milk production in nursing mothers.

The most common use of fennel, however, is in treating overactive intestinal motility resulting in cramps or colic. Fennel makes an extremely enjoyable tea. In fact, in addition to its culinary uses, fennel is also used as a flavoring agent in absinthe and other liquors.

You can see that there is considerable similarity between the herbs of a group. Yet while sharing certain characteristics, each herb has a particular strong point. For me, these two principles underline the validity of the basic approach of presenting herbs within groups.

I am convinced that one can build a useful fund of herbal knowledge, more than sufficient to treat the majority of illnesses encountered, by understanding the properties of the herb groups and becoming familiar with a few herbs in each.

Bitter Digestives

*J*ust as the aromatics are used for digestive disorders when warming is required, the bitter digestives are favored when a cooling effect is more beneficial. It is convenient to divide digestive effects into two categories: those that stimulate digestive processes and those that relieve digestive symptoms. Looked at in this way, the strong point of bitter digestives is that they aid digestion, favorably influencing the absorption and uptake of food, while the antispasmodics (to be discussed later) are most often employed to calm digestive distress.

While in classical herbal thinking the cooling herbs are believed to deplete the body's reserves, the bitter digestives are an exception. Instead they are believed to take body heat and convert it into nourishment and energy. Bitters are considered to be tonic herbs and can be used in patients who are debilitated or suffering from a chronic disease where digestive problems appear to be a contributing factor.

All of the bitters have a positive effect on every aspect of digestion. They tend to increase the appetite, enhance the movement of food in the gut, and increase the secretion of digestive enzymes. The net result is an increase in available nourishment and an increase in the body's vital energy.

The bitters are also beneficial in the treatment of diseases of the gallbladder and liver. Some members of the group (cholagogues) are said to exert a pronounced effect on the secretion of bile into the intestine and have curative properties regarding liver disease. These will be pointed out later in the chapter.

GENTIAN

Gentian is possibly the most widely used bitter. In fact, it is the classic bitter herb and could well be used as the basis of any formula requiring a bitter principle. Gentian extract has been shown to stimulate appetite.

It also promotes secretion of enzymes from the stomach, pancreas, and intestine, thus facilitating digestion. It is indicated whenever a digestive aid is needed, particularly when a cooling effect is desired. Gentian is also believed to have anti-inflammatory properties and has been used to treat gout.

MILK THISTLE

Milk thistle shares the usual properties of the group as a digestive stimulant. In modern herbal usage, however, its action on the liver has received the most attention. A great deal of research in Europe has shown that this herb improves liver function, protecting the liver from chemical injury and even enhancing the formation of new liver cells. It has therefore become the primary liver tonic in Europe.

Industrialization has unfortunately unleashed a modern epidemic of pollution. Many occupational toxins must be broken down by the liver, thus its burden has been magnified in recent times. Milk thistle has emerged as the major liver tonic in use today. If you are using tablets or capsules, the usual dose is two, twice a day—but, as always, check the manufacturer's recommendations.

DANDELION

Long maligned by people seeking perfect lawns, dandelion is a widely used herb with several noteworthy properties. As a digestive aid it is believed to exert a particularly potent effect on the gallbladder by stimulating the secretion of bile. Dandelion increases bile secretion by 50 percent, and studies have confirmed enhanced secretion of bilirubin only minutes after administration.

Dandelion is also believed to exert a curative effect on the liver and is thus commonly used in liver ailments. It has also been used for gallstones and urinary tract stones. In addition, dandelion also acts as a diuretic (ridding the body of excessive water) and is believed to be useful for kidney problems.

Some consider dandelion to be beneficial in the treatment of swollen breasts. Dandelion is also used in the treatment of arthritic problems and thus is claimed to have anti-inflammatory properties. It is best thought of as a bitter digestive particularly useful for problems of the gallbladder, liver, and kidneys.

YELLOW DOCK

Yellow dock, in addition to its expected properties as a bitter, also acts as a blood cleanser. Most specifically it is indicated when skin or joint problems (such as eczema, psoriasis, or arthritis) coexist with evidence of liver disease or digestive dysfunction (abnormal bowel movements, excessive gas, bloating, and so on). In practice, however, it is often used as a blood purifier for skin and joint problems in the absence of digestive difficulties. It also has laxative properties and is used as an aid in elimination.

Yellow dock is most useful in conditions calling for a digestive aid with cleansing properties. (In herbal traditions, many disorders, particularly those affecting joints or skin, are considered to benefit from a general cleansing because they are thought to result from the accumulation of toxins. This will be discussed in detail in Chapter 13, which deals specifically with the cleansing herbs.

GOLDENSEAL

Goldenseal is considered a potent bitter herb sharing the usual properties of others in the group. What makes it noteworthy is its beneficial effect on the mucous membranes, the tissues that make up the inner lining of the body. In this regard its major use is for inflammation or ulceration of the upper gastrointestinal tract, especially the esophagus, stomach, or duodenum.

It can also be used as a mouthwash or douche and is considered the most potent restorative herb for mucous membranes.

With fast foods, meals on the run, and skipped meals so commonplace, a digestive adjunct would seem to form a reasonable basis for any tonic mixture. Given the fast-paced, deadline-driven schedules that most of us face, along with the tensions and pressures of everyday life, a cooling, calming bitter herb seems most appropriate. For modern times the bitter digestives may be the ideal tonic.

Vasodilators

*T*he vasodilators are the classic warming herbs. In the era before antibiotics, these drugs were the mainstay of the treatment of infectious diseases. They were used to help maintain a fever at optimal level, provide a cleansing sweat, and even to induce a therapeutic fever when it was believed that this was warranted.

In modern herbal therapeutics, these drugs are used primarily as warming agents (a character shared by all drugs of this group) and to open up the circulation when this is impaired. The warming herbs are indicated in all cases characterized by a sluggish response to disease. The patient who is lethargic, easily fatigued, and shows decreased vitality and a depressed level of bodily functions will benefit from herbs of this class. They are obviously indicated in all cases where the patient has the sensation of feeling cold or chilled.

GINGER

Ginger is a warming drug with several effects that make it a useful herb with widespread application. It provokes a cleansing sweat (diaphoretic effect), and this effect, along with its properties as an expectorant, make it an ideal herb for bronchial infections. Likewise, it is very widely used in mild gastrointestinal infections because its diaphoretic effect, combined with its penchant to control nausea, vomiting, and diarrhea, make it a sound choice.

A study published in the prestigious British medical journal *The Lancet* found ginger more effective than Dramamine in preventing nausea associated with motion sickness. It has vasodilating properties and is widely used to increase circulation to the extremities when this is impaired. Powdered dry ginger is very effective; it needs to be used only twice daily.

In short, ginger is most often used when a warming agent is required, especially when its expectorant properties or its calming effect on the gastrointestinal system would be beneficial, or as an aid to increase peripheral circulation.

CAYENNE

Cayenne can be used as a warming agent in virtually all prescriptions that require one. It increases delivery of the herb mixture throughout the body and acts as an enhancer for the other herbs present. It can be used as a digestive aid and has anti-inflammatory properties that warrant its use for both headache and arthritis.

Cluster headaches, which are severe and occur nightly for weeks at a time, may be particularly responsive to cayenne. It should be considered as a general aid to circulation and as an adjunct in prescriptions requiring heating.

HAWTHORN

Hawthorn is an herb with a long history of use as a circulatory aid. Not only does it improve the general circulation, but it is also used for impaired circulation to the extremities, manifested either by pain upon walking or by discomfort or discoloration on exposure to cold. It has also been used for venous problems, including varicose veins. In addition, hawthorn has been used for hypertension.

But its greatest potential benefit is in the treatment of coronary artery disease, the leading cause of death today. It has a multitude of effects, all of which benefit the patient with coronary heart disease. Hawthorn has a direct vasodilating effect on the coronary arteries, increasing the supply of blood to the heart. It tends to lower the heart rate and helps the heart maintain a regular cardiac rhythm. It is said to lower cholesterol levels and has a mild sedating effect, which is often beneficial for patients with heart disease. Lastly, hawthorn tends to increase the strength of contractions of the heart muscle. It is therefore, the premier herb in use today for cardiac difficulties. It should be considered in the treatment of cardiac problems or whenever circulation is impaired.

Freeze-dried hawthorn in capsule form is available. The dose is one or two capsules, two to four times a day.

GINKGO

Ginkgo is a mainstay of European herbal therapy. Its beneficial effects are related primarily to its activity as a vasodilator. It has been demonstrated to increase circulation to the brain as well as to the extremities. In one study, 75 percent of elderly patients with cerebral insufficiency (decreased blood supply to the brain) showed improvement in flow with ginkgo. More remarkably, a recent English study showed an improvement in the memory of young women as well.

Thus ginkgo appears to increase memory, ability to concentrate, and cognitive functioning throughout life. It also increases peripheral blood flow and can be used in all cases of poor circulation. Cases of phlebitis and varicose veins may likewise benefit from therapy with this herb.

Ginkgo decreases the "stickiness" of platelets so that they are less likely to clump and form a clot with a resultant stroke or heart attack. In addition to all of these beneficial effects on circulation, it is also believed to benefit patients with tinnitis (ringing in the ears) and those with depression. Ginkgo is deservedly the most widely prescribed herb in Germany, where it is used primarily for its beneficial circulatory effects, but its usefulness in tinnitis and depression should also be borne in mind.

FEVERFEW

Feverfew has had a long history of use for headache. Articles published in Great Britain in the 1970s and 1980s have confirmed its effectiveness. It was found to cure migraine and to prevent its occurrence when taken prophylactically. (Note: Some experts say that it is parthenolide, a natural chemical found in feverfew and some other plants, that rids the person of a migraine, but not all feverfew preparations include this substance.)

Feverfew has also demonstrated anti-inflammatory effects and has been used in arthritic conditions.

Feverfew grows in many areas of the world and grows wild in some areas of the northeast coast of the United States.

GARLIC

Garlic has multiple uses: it has been employed in the treatment of cancer, arthritis, liver disease, and many other maladies. We will concentrate on those areas of greatest benefit and utility.

Garlic strengthens the body's defenses, making it better able to protect itself against pathogens (disease-causing organisms); thus it is useful in infections in general, particularly those affecting the lung and gut. Like ginger, garlic has warming expectorant properties resulting in a drying up and elimination of excessive mucous.

The volatile oils in garlic are excreted via exhalation and exert a sterilizing effect on the lungs. Thus garlic is useful for all lung infections and has been used with good results in the treatment of asthma. Garlic also has an anti-infectious effect on disease-causing organisms in the gut, and this—along with its trait as a digestive aid—make it an herb of choice for gastrointestinal infections.

It also is a useful herb to prevent or treat heart disease. Garlic is said to lower cholesterol levels and decrease blood clotting while acting as a vasodilator and counteracting atherosclerosis. I do not recommend "deodorized" garlic because we simply do not know whether the health benefits of this herb are dependent on its odoriferous components.

Though it is hard to pin garlic down to a few effects, it is perhaps most useful for lung and gastrointestinal infections, as a digestive aid, and finally for heart disease, particularly as a preventative.

Vasodilators and Circulation

The vasodilators are warming in temperament and exert their major effect on the circulation. They have been used for peripheral arterial disease, venous disease, and to improve the coronary circulation (notably hawthorn).

Ginkgo is considered to be especially beneficial to the cerebral circulation. Some herbs in this class (ginger and garlic) are particularly useful for infections of the lung and digestive tract. Cayenne tends to increase the efficiency of all herbs in a mixture when a warming influence is required.

Consequently, even though these herbs are rarely used in their ancient roles as diaphoretics or fever inducers, they remain an integral part of the herbal armamentarium.

Sedatives and Antispasmodics

*7*he sedatives and antispasmodics have a calming or soothing effect. Although the major action of each drug in this class will be either in the psychological (sedative) area, or on the body (antispasmodic), it should be understood that all the herbs discussed in this section have both qualities even though we may be highlighting one.

Like the bitter digestives, these drugs are cooling in nature and, like the bitters, they are much needed in our highly stressed and pressured era. The sedatives and antispasmodics are generally indicated in patients who exhibit excitability, nervousness, tension, and overactivity—either mentally, physically, or both.

VALERIAN

Valerian is the first herb in this group that we will consider. It has been used successfully for many conditions believed to have a nervous or anxious component, especially when associated with an element of muscle spasm, since it does have antispasmodic qualities.

It is very useful for headache, especially tension cephalalgia (headache caused by anxiety or tension). Valerian finds its greatest utility as a valued tranquilizer. Unlike most prescribed tranquilizers, it has no additive effect with alcohol and no addictive potential. It can be considered a nonsedating tranquilizer. Thus while promoting a calm and relaxed mood, valerian will not negatively affect level of arousal or alertness. Some scientists, however, believe that valerian does have depressant properties and would caution against long-term use.

Valerian is also highly regarded as a mild sleep aid, and its effectiveness has been proven in clinical studies where the time required to fall asleep was decreased in patients using the herb. In addition, there was no morning "hangover" and, in fact, morning sleepiness was decreased (in keeping with its nonsedating character).

Valerian is particularly useful in the treatment of behavioral and learning problems in childhood, as discussed in Chapter 26. An authentic tranquilizer, valerian is also an extremely useful sleep aid and a primary drug in the treatment of common tension headache.

PASSIONFLOWER

Passionflower is also a foremost natural tranquilizer. Since it also acts as a muscle relaxant, it is an excellent herb for nervous conditions associated with muscle spasm and restlessness, and also has been used effectively for tension headache. In comparison to valerian, it is used generally in the more severe cases of anxiety or psychological distress.

It is quite useful for insomnia, but it should be borne in mind that, unlike valerian, passionflower has a sedative effect and can cause drowsiness. Thus passionflower may be considered, like valerian, to be a natural tranquilizer but perhaps to be used mainly in more serious cases.

CHAMOMILE

Chamomile is used most specifically in two settings. It is employed as an antispasmodic and is thus indicated in the treatment of stomach cramps, intestinal spasms, colic, or excessive gas.

A second major indication for chamomile is disordered gynecological function, and it has been used by women for centuries to treat menstrual difficulties including painful periods and symptoms of menopause. Chamomile has also been used for mastitis (inflammation and pain in the breast) with good results. Like the herbs mentioned above, it can be applied to nervous or anxious conditions. Chamomile has been used for headache and insomnia as well.

In the laboratory, animals given chamomile appear less anxious, quite relaxed, and perhaps less inquisitive. Coordination and motor function are not impaired. Chamomile's wide usage is therefore most justified since it safely helps to pacify us from so many of the troubles associated with modern life. It should be considered whenever one requires a gentle relaxant, an herb to calm the gut, or treatment of gynecological problems. It is especially enjoyable when taken as tea.

PEPPERMINT

Peppermint shares in the antispasmodic and relaxant qualities of other herbs in the class. It is used for nervousness, insomnia, and headache. It is a useful herb to relieve gas, colic, and intestinal spasm associated with anxiety or mild gastrointestinal infection. Peppermint has been shown to have a relaxing effect on the smooth muscle of the gut, confirming its effectiveness as an antispasmodic.

But because peppermint can relax the sphincter muscle between the stomach and the esophagus, it can worsen symptoms of hiatal hernia and acid reflux (acid moving backward) into the esophagus.

Peppermint is an excellent treatment for nausea and vomiting. This feature, combined with the fact that it is by far the best-tasting herb of the group, ensures its popularity in herbal therapy. Peppermint is available in enteric coated capsules to protect the stomach.

HOPS

Hops have marked sedative properties and are a time-honored cure for insomnia. Sleeping on hops pillows (made by putting hops in a pillow and drizzling with alcohol) is an alternative cure for sleeplessness. Hops are also commonly used simply for their calming effect on the nervous system and in cases of restlessness.

The major use of hops is for their muscle relaxant properties. Hops appear to exert this effect most conspicuously on the bowel, and they are therefore a most useful drug in states of colitis or irritable bowel syndrome. They help relieve excessive gas, cramps, and diarrhea. Hops therefore are useful as a sedative generally and as an antispasmodic, particularly in disorders of the colon, where they prove to be a highly beneficial herbal remedy.

We have just considered a group of herbs with a calming effect upon both the body and the spirit. They are drugs whose utility cannot be questioned in our hectic, frantic times. But a word of caution is in order. When discussing the temperament of herbal remedies, we cited cooling drugs as somehow taking away some of the vital energy of life. All the drugs in this class are cooling in nature.

When taken appropriately they will be found to be efficacious and beneficial. The concept of balance or harmony is important, and at times calming herbal medications are necessary to reestablish a sense of wholeness.

However, one should not ignore the calming and pacifying qualities of a short period of rest, a walk in the park, enjoying some music or art, quality time with a dear friend or loved one, or a period of prayer or meditation. These have medicinal value as well and should never be slighted. They are present in any complete prescription for wellness.

CHAPTER 11

Diuretics

Since most plants contain substances that must be excreted by the kidneys, almost all plants could be said to have some diuretic properties. In this chapter I will concentrate on those herbs that have a marked effect on urine volume and that have therefore earned a place in the herbal apothecary as diuretic herbs.

Nearly all prescription diuretics tend to cause a loss of potassium in the urine, thus depleting the body's potassium stores. When one is using herbal diuretics, this is seldom a problem since their action tends to be milder. Also, most plant sources are rich in potassium, helping to replenish what is lost.

As mentioned earlier, the herbalist emphasizes the importance of elimination, believing that the accumulation of toxins plays a role in many illnesses and contributes much to infirmity and disease. It is not my goal here to defend or condemn this viewpoint. However, while it is true that this belief may sound old-fashioned, unscientific, or naïve, it should be remembered that modern medicine is quite unable to supply a clear-cut cause or etiology for many of the diseases it purports to treat.

Thus, although the cleansing action of herbal diuretics is often called on to improve "toxic" skin conditions or many arthritic problems, rather than smiling at the apparent simple-mindedness of this approach, we should remember that it is based on centuries of accumulated clinical experience. We will now consider some widely used diuretics, as always trying to emphasize those characteristics that are singular to each herb.

PARSLEY

Parsley is a rather potent herbal diuretic. Since it is quite high in potassium, one need not worry much about potassium loss in the urine. It has been used in the treatment of hypertension, with favorable results published in the *American Journal of Chinese Medicine*.

Parsley also has a reputation for helping rid the body of metabolic waste products and thus has a strong tradition of use in arthritic conditions.

An added benefit of parsley is that it relieves intestinal spasm and gas. It is used effectively for premenstrual syndrome and also has been credited with bringing on delayed menses. Parsley should be considered in all conditions where a significant diuretic is indicated, and it is believed to be useful in herbal mixtures for arthritis.

UVA URSI

Uva ursi has urinary antiseptic properties and has been used quite effectively in the treatment of urinary tract infections. It has diuretic properties as well. The body converts a constituent of uva ursi to hydroquinone, a urinary tract disinfectant. Uva ursi is also soothing to the urinary tract, helping to relieve the painful symptoms of infection in this system. Thus, uva ursi is a soothing diuretic with antiseptic properties in the urinary tract.

HORSETAIL

Horsetail is a useful diuretic believed to be particularly effective in states of fluid retention due to hormonal causes, especially when associated with menopause. It is reputed to increase absorption of calcium, an important consideration in postmenopausal women. Horsetail has also been used for hypertension.

It is used for urinary tract infections and is also considered a useful cleanser, particularly for arthritic and skin problems. Consequently, one major role of horsetail is to counteract fluid retention, especially in women who particularly benefit from increased calcium absorption. Horsetail is also used as a diuretic with cleansing properties.

CHAPTER 12

Cold Medications and Expectorants

*T*he expectorants all share a common quality; they promote cough and aid in the removal of foreign material from the lungs. Again, this fits in with the general herbal goal of elimination. When one considers that bronchitis generally consists of a viral or bacterial infection in the bronchial tubes or is due to irritating foreign material, the good sense of elimination as a basic strategy becomes obvious. Removal of the insulting pathogen should form the basis of any therapeutic regimen

However, while all expectorants encourage the removal of material from the lungs, they are separated into two groups related to their effects on mucous or phlegm. In contemporary parlance, one group is indicated for a dry cough (the moistening expectorants) and the second group is utilized generally when the cough is productive (the drying expectorants).

THYME

Thyme is an herb with great utility for respiratory problems. It is particularly useful in the asthmatic, since it relaxes spasm in the airways, thus easing respiratory distress. Its moistening quality loosens up, or decreases the viscosity of, respiratory secretions and then stimulates the bronchi, encouraging expectoration. In addition, it also helps sterilize the lung and is thus advantageous in any respiratory infection.

Brian M. Lawrence, Ph.D., editor of the *Journal of Essential Oil Research* and a noted research scientist, affirms that thymol has "well-known bacterial and antifungal properties," explaining its inclusion in over-the-counter products like Vicks VapoRub ointment and Listerine mouthwash. Thyme is therefore a front-line herb for respiratory infections where phlegm is scant or thick, and it is particularly indicated in asthmatics.

ELECAMPANE

Elecampane is used when respiratory infection is associated with profuse mucous secretion. It dries up excessive phlegm and stimulates its removal via the bronchial tubes. Like thyme, it has antibacterial properties, and it is well utilized in respiratory infections.

In fact, elecampane was used in the treatment of bronchitis and other respiratory problems by Ayurvedic physicians in India, as well as by the ancient Chinese. It also promotes bile flow and has been used in the treatment of liver distress. Its greatest utility, however, is in respiratory infections with overabundant secretions.

MA HUANG

Ma huang is a vasodilating herb, but its major utility derives from its effects on the respiratory tract. Thus, in deference to its most common usage, I have opted to consider this herb in the expectorant group. It causes a relaxation of the airways and drying of secretions and is therefore a mainstay in the treatment of respiratory tract infections.

Ma huang is useful in the treatment of asthma as well, relaxing spasm in the bronchial tree, and has been used with good effect in other airway hypersensitivity syndromes like hay fever. Ma huang is also believed to be of benefit in flulike states and for treating symptoms of the common cold.

Because of its potential hypertensive effect, it should not be used by patients with high blood pressure, except with medical supervision. It also stimulates the central nervous system and should be avoided by those sensitive to such effects. This forms the basis for its use in herbal weight loss remedies. In summary, then, ma huang provides great benefit to the respiratory tract; it is useful in a wide variety of conditions including asthma, hay fever, bronchitis, and even treats symptoms of cold or flu.

Of the herbs mentioned in other chapters, three in particular have sufficient expectorant properties to make them useful enough to be included in the expectorant group.

Angelica has diaphoretic and expectorant properties and is discussed with the aromatic digestives.

Garlic is also widely used in respiratory infections and is discussed with the vasodilators. Angelica and garlic, like elecampane, are drying expectorants.

Licorice is a tonic herb that has significant activity as a moistening expectorant.

WILD BLACK CHERRY AND WILD CHERRY BARK

Wild black cherry and wild cherry bark are not expectorants and therefore do not aid in the elimination of foreign material from the lungs. In fact, their effect is quite the opposite. They are antitussives and act to suppress the cough reflex; they should only be considered when cough is debilitating.

Cleansing Herbs—Getting Rid of Toxins

These important herbs are believed to cleanse the body but without having an obvious effect on elimination. Their primary use is in the treatment of inflammatory conditions; that is, illnesses characterized by heat, redness, and swelling. Many of these conditions occur on the skin, and these herbs are said to benefit patients with eczema, psoriasis, boils, carbuncles, and other skin eruptions. This group of herbs is also favored in the treatment of arthritic conditions.

It is of interest that the herbalist chooses to treat these diseases with herbs that are believed to cleanse or purify. The inflammatory response is respected; as always the reaction of the body is held in high esteem. The Western, scientific approach of employing drugs to blunt that response (anti-inflammatories) is considered by the herbalist to afford only symptomatic relief and to ignore the basic problem. Again, my role here is not to take sides in the dispute but simply to point out the difference in orientation.

The various herbs in this group and their particular strengths will be discussed individually. Some are believed to cleanse the blood, while others cleanse the lymphatic system (for example the lymph glands in the neck.) Still others are believed to be general cleansers that will eliminate toxins by whatever appears to be the most efficient route.

There is little scientific evidence supporting the claims that these herbs work in this manner, but most herbalists are not overly concerned about this. Centuries of efficacious use have shown that these herbs do work in certain inflammatory conditions. "Blood cleanser" may not stand up to rigid scientific scrutiny, but it may not mean the same thing to the herbalist and the pathologist. Perhaps the terms should not be taken too literally.

BURDOCK

Burdock is regarded as probably the single most active blood purifier. It is said to neutralize poisons and evacuate them from the body. It is used in a variety of inflammatory skin conditions including eczema, psoriasis, canker sores, boils, and carbuncles. Burdock is also widely used in the treatment of arthritis and rheumatism. In addition, it possesses diuretic properties. Burdock should be considered an unparalleled blood cleanser for use in skin and arthritic conditions.

NETTLE

Nettle is a detoxifying agent used in inflammatory conditions, particularly arthritic (but also skin) problems. Two of its other properties are believed to add to its effectiveness for this purpose: it is a diuretic and is believed to aid in the excretion of metabolic wastes (which are believed to accumulate in these diseases), and it increases the circulation to further the body's inflammatory response.

Nettle is also used in premenstrual syndrome and promotes the breast milk flow in nursing mothers. It also lowers the blood sugar level in diabetics. We will consider nettle mainly as a prime cleansing herb for use in arthritic conditions.

DEVIL'S CLAW

Devil's claw is a relatively recent addition to the herbal pharmacopoeia in the United States but has been used in Europe for close to 300 years and even longer in its native Africa. It is used to reduce inflammation and pain in arthritis and myositis (muscle pain).

Devil's claw is used primarily in the treatment of oral problems and is used for infections and inflammations of the mouth and throat. It can also be used as a douche in vaginal irritations. This herb is believed to have direct antiseptic action, to support the body's defenses against infection, and to be reparative to damaged tissue, thus promoting healing and renewal.

MYRRH

Myrrh has a long and esteemed tradition in herbal medicine. Its benefits are alluded to in both the Old and New Testaments of the Bible. Overall, myrrh finds its greatest utility when used topically for infirmities of the mucous membranes, especially the mouth and throat.

ECHINACEA

Echinacea is an herb of North American origin. It was, in fact, the most commonly used plant by North American Indians. Word of its effectiveness spread, and it is now highly regarded in Europe as well. It is believed to be a blood purifier and is used in that role for boils, carbuncles, acne, psoriasis, and eczema.

Recent research, however, has unearthed more far-reaching effects. Studies indicate that echinacea helps to maintain the body's natural barriers that prevent spread of infection. It is believed to have antiseptic and antiviral properties, stimulating the white blood cells that fight infection. The activity of macrophages (cells that fight infection by ingesting foreign materials) is enhanced by echinacea.

Echinacea has been used to help restore normal immune function and is being studied in the treatment of AIDS. It has been employed in the treatment of cancer, where its beneficial effects are also probably mediated by enhancing the immune mechanism, and thus it is considered beneficial to the lymphatic system.

This is an herb with a multitude of effects that secure its valued place in contemporary herbalism. Echinacea should be taken into account in treating any infectious condition or any skin condition that would benefit from a blood cleanser.

The cleansing herbs find multiple uses in modern herbal therapeutics. An herbal mixture for arthritic or rheumatic pain would benefit from the addition of one of these herbs (particularly consider nettle or devil's claw). Common toxic skin conditions are often seen to benefit from a course of treatment with burdock. Echinacea finds widespread use today, being valued in the treatment of virtually all infections, including the common cold. These are abundantly useful herbs in a variety of conditions and demonstrate unparalleled safety.

CHAPTER 14

Tonic Herbs—
Energizing Yourself

*T*he tonic herbs are believed to have a rejuvenating or restorative effect on an organ system or on the body as a whole. They reinvigorate the body, replacing what has been lost as a result of illness or stress. Those who are weak by disposition are strengthened by the use of tonic herbs. These medicines are believed to be supporting and nourishing, bringing us to our own personal, individual state of maximal vitality and vigor.

In certain herbal traditions these drugs are also considered to be balancing in nature, helping to establish a state of equilibrium and moving us to a point of focus or clarity. This is believed to be possible both in the psychological sphere (where the same herb may be capable of moderating either mania or melancholy) or physically (where an herb may be capable of either stimulating deficient hormonal production or ameliorating its excessive manufacture).

Ancient cultures believe that wisdom, harmony, or balance can spill over, resulting in humans being at peace in the spiritual realm as well. People are a composite of physical, mental, emotional, and spiritual spheres, and there is an intimate interaction among them. In alternative medicine, good health is the result of a person being in harmony on all four levels. The tonic herbs, more than any others, are believed to aid in this all-encompassing quest.

The first three herbs have their primary effect on the nervous system—on the mood, disposition, or temper. Although this emphasis on one area is contrary to the general plan of this book, it is done here intentionally. For it is this area that seems the most in disarray today. When considering the concepts of harmony or balance, you must inevitably also be concerned with the psyche. Until we have reached a level of order, symmetry, and peace where mind and spirit converge, then true wellness is only an illusion.

OATS

Oats have long been employed in the treatment of nervous system disorders. They are used for shingles, multiple sclerosis, neuritis, and neuralgia, as well as for psychological disorders. They are considered particularly effective in countering depression and melancholia. Oats are thus believed to be a restorative to the nervous system both physically and psychologically.

SAINT-JOHN'S-WORT

Saint-John's-wort is a tonic with a definite calming effect. It is extremely useful in states of anxiety or emotional tension; unlike many psychoactive drugs, it appears to be free of side effects. It has been used for depression and insomnia. Its muscle relaxant properties make it useful for bed-wetting, irritable colon syndrome, painful menses, and menopausal symptoms. Saint-John's-wort should be considered a tonic restorative to the nervous system with calming and relaxing actions.

GOTU KOLA

Gotu kola has been used in Asian medicine for over two thousand years. In the West it has become known primarily as a relaxing nerve tonic. Its advocates claim that it improves cognitive functions of the brain and increases memory. Indian herbal literature contains numerous citations attesting to the positive effect of gotu kola on intelligence.

Gotu kola has been used for phlebitis because it reportedly decreases pain and swelling of the affected vein. Gotu kola is used here primarily as a relaxing nerve tonic that may improve cerebral processes and memory.

LICORICE

Licorice is not only a popular flavoring for candies but also one of the most widely used medicinal plants in the world. It can be used as a gentle laxative and has a long history of use for inflammation of the stomach and peptic ulcers, where it is said to decrease production of acid and supply a protective coating mucus. It also increases mucus production in the lungs and is a useful expectorant.

Licorice stimulates the production of the hormone cortisone, and this in concert with its expectorant properties makes it an ideal drug for asthma. Its cortisone-stimulating effect explains its time-honored use in the treatment of arthritis as well.

A word of caution: in stimulating cortisone production, licorice also increases production of another hormone (aldosterone) that can cause high blood pressure and loss of potassium. Generally, this is only seen with high doses over long periods.

Glycyrrhetic acid, found in high concentration in licorice, has significant anti-inflammatory effects and also contributes to its successful use in arthritic conditions. In addition to these tangible effects, licorice is considered to be a harmony remedy in the Chinese tradition, again harkening back to the notion of ill health as being the end result of a lack of balance in mind, body, or spirit. Therefore, licorice is considered a cooling tonic or harmony herb, also beneficial in the treatment of ulcers, asthma or bronchitis, and arthritis.

The tonic herbs are among the most widely used and valued medicines in our day. Perhaps their popularity is simply another manifestation of how disjointed and unbalanced modern man has become. Incorporation of a regular period of relaxation, meditation, or appreciation of art, literature, or music might well be considered an additional essential prescription for our time.

Chinese Tonic Herbs

*W*hile the concepts of hot and cold as considered in Western herbal medicine are easily presented and understood, Asian ideas allow for no such simple interpretation. For example, in Chinese thought, yin and yang are the complementary characteristics of all reality. However, to simply consider yin to be the passive or female quality and yang to be the active or male quality not only does a great disservice to the concepts of male and female, but also profoundly distorts the original Chinese concepts.

Yin and yang encompass all pairs of opposites. Right and left, black and white, large and small are all examples of yin and yang. To complicate things further, yang is lower and yin is higher. Yet the branch of a tree is yin (higher) compared to the ground but yang (lower) compared to the sky. Reality consists of the coexistence, interplay, and harmony of all possible opposites. Similarly, the notions behind traditional Chinese physiology—notions that deal with change, flux, and energy—are complex and elegant but require a mode of thinking quite alien to Western patterns. I will therefore simply discuss several of the most commonly used Chinese herbs and their indications. As with the Western tonic herbs, these herbs are believed to be balancing and revitalizing, particularly useful for those whose energy levels are depleted and quite applicable therefore for modern times.

GINSENG

Considering its great esteem in China and popularity in the West, ginseng will be discussed first. In China, ginseng has been used virtually as a panacea and has been utilized in practically all ailments for thousands of years. It is believed to increase energy, to fortify the mental, physical, and emotional levels, and is believed to be particularly applicable in times of stress.

An interesting, well-designed, and well-executed study involving nurses found that the group taking ginseng scored higher in the areas of mental and physical performance, mood, and overall competence. Numerous studies have confirmed these findings.

Ginseng is considered to be mildly stimulating to the nervous system. It has a reputation as a Chinese "fountain of youth," helping to forestall aging and enhance youthful vigor. It is thought to have a balancing or equalizing effect on mental and physical processes and is claimed to have aphrodisiac qualities.

Ginseng is a highly favored herb believed to be most useful in times of stress, as an antiaging herb, and in promoting physical and mental harmony. A standardized extract is now widely available.

DONG QUAI

Dong quai has been hailed as "female ginseng" because of its great utility in the treatment of gynecological problems, including painful or irregular periods, absent menses, or pelvic infections. It is believed to be useful for premenstrual syndrome and menopausal symptoms as well. Dong quai has a high concentration of phytoestrogens (plant substances with estrogenic activity). It has been demonstrated to have a relaxing effect on the smooth muscle of the uterus and has both pain relieving and tranquilizing effects as well.

Dong quai is believed to be an invigorating tonic herb, restoring strength to those who are significantly deficient. It is also recommended for use in heart disease, where it is said to open up the arteries, lower cholesterol, and maintain a normal cardiac rhythm. It is also believed to increase circulation to the extremities. Dong quai is thus considered a revitalizing herb, an herb with great utility in a host of female reproductive difficulties, and an aid in heart disease.

FENUGREEK

Fenugreek is a time-honored Asian and Western remedy dating back to the era of Hippocrates. It has been used for those suffering from chronic conditions such as tuberculosis and in the recovery phase from substantial illnesses. It has been used as an aphrodisiac and to stimulate production of breast milk. Fenugreek has been confirmed to lower blood sugar level in diabetics (an effect similar to insulin). Today fenugreek is considered mainly as a restorative herb to increase vital energy, to help combat illness, or to restore depleted energy reserves during convalescence.

ASTRAGALUS

Astragalus is a popular herb among the Chinese. It is believed to be an energizing remedy and is most favored by those who are physically active. It is also considered to be a tonic for the immune system, helping to fortify the body's defenses against infection. Favorable effects in this regard were reported in *Cancer,* the prestigious publication of the American Cancer Society. It is most used today as an energizing tonic by the physically active, to protect the body against infection, and in the treatment of cancer.

We have considered four of the most popular and widely used Chinese herbs, giving concrete examples of their most common usages and reputed properties. Although I have omitted specific discussion of Chinese physiology, there is a Chinese concept that must be cited. In ancient Chinese medicine, health is viewed holistically. The interrelationship between mind and body has always been understood; there is nothing akin to the Western separation of the two spheres.

In Chinese (and all nonmodern) medicine, a human is not compartmentalized but is one. As a result, this mindset essentially considers any medical system that segregates a person into his component biological systems, each to be treated by a different specialist, to be doomed at the outset. The human is a whole; he cannot be compartmentalized physically and certainly should not be compartmentalized when being administered to. We become ill when there is an element of disorder in our whole life pattern. It is only by bringing all of oneself together, into balance, and achieving a state of harmony and symmetry that we again can become well.

It is in this most ethereal realm, most distant from physiologic oversimplification and most removed from scientific scrutiny, that the tonic herbs may well exert their most enduring effects. Licorice in the Western sphere and ginseng in the Chinese tradition are believed to be most active here.

Male Hormonal Herbs

*T*he following herbs, although applicable to both sexes, have major uses for men, particularly in the realm of declining or weakening sexual function and general deterioration and infirmity associated with the aging process. Given their reputed properties, it is not surprising that they are among the most widely used herbal products. In men these herbs are often used concurrently. They will be considered as a group in one chapter for two reasons: first, they do have a noted effect on male dysfunction, and second, there is a group of herbs whose greatest utility is related to female difficulties (see Chapter 17) and these herbs seemed to be the male equivalent.

One must, however, always bear in mind that all herbs have multiple effects, and these are no exception. They have qualities that are beneficial to both sexes and are frequently used with good effect in women. Women should not avoid these herbs simply because they are discussed in this chapter. They will not cause any untoward hormonal effects when used by women (excess body hair, voice change, and so on).

DAMIANA

Damiana is considered a tonic herb for the nervous system and has been used with particular effectiveness in the treatment of headache, anxiety, and depression. It is believed to lead to a feeling of contentment. Its scientific name, *Turnera aphrodisiaca,* gives a clue to its other major role: it is believed to be a sexual stimulant and to enhance sexual performance in both sexes, especially in men. It is said to be particularly effective when sexual inadequacies have a psychological underpinning.

SEVEN BARKS

Seven barks is used in both sexes as a diuretic and in the treatment of stones in the urinary tract. It is believed to ward off the physical and mental decline of aging in males.

SAW PALMETTO

Saw palmetto is believed (like seven barks) to prevent senescence and weakness in men of advancing years. It is thought to be useful for urinary tract infections in both sexes and has been used for non-cancerous enlargement of the prostate (benign prostatic hypertrophy, or BPH).

A well-designed study showed a marked improvement in symptoms of prostate enlargement in those patients given extract of saw palmetto. These patients had a decrease in nighttime urination of about 50 percent and a 50 percent increase in the force of urine flow. These findings have been confirmed by other investigators. Saw palmetto is also believed by some to have aphrodisiac qualities, again more prominently noticed in the male. It has been used as a tonic during periods of convalescence.

Again, placing these herbs in a chapter for men relates to a constellation of effects. These effects, however, are not the sum total of their actions; therefore appropriate use of these herbs in women is not to be discouraged.

Female Hormonal Herbs

*7*he herbs addressed in this chapter share a single characteristic: a predominant effect on female reproductive function. However, a similar caveat should be stated here as in the preceding chapter. Although these herbs may have developed a strong reputation based on their effectiveness in this area, like all herbs they have multiple actions. Some of these may be advantageous to men as well as women. Thus these herbs should not be considered for female use only, and men should not be reluctant to take advantage of them when indicated.

DONG QUAI

Dong quai, which was discussed in Chapter 15, is also a foremost remedy for many female problems. It is believed to normalize the menstrual cycle, reinstating a menstrual flow or regulating the menses when they are excessive or irregular. It has been used for inflammation and infection in this area and is claimed to be useful in the treatment of premenstrual syndrome and menopausal symptoms. It is also used both as a tonic herb and for heart disease as well. For our consideration here, however, dong quai can be considered an herb useful for virtually all female gynecological problems. The usual dose is two capsules twice a day. For menstrual problems you should give it at least a two-month trial before giving up on it.

SQUAW VINE

Squaw vine is a Native American Indian remedy. It has traditionally been taken during the last several weeks of pregnancy to make childbirth easier. Today it is commonly employed for menstrual cramps. It possesses diuretic properties that may be helpful to counteract fluid retention related to menses. It has also been used for nervous exhaustion in both sexes. Squaw vine is thus primarily to be considered as an herb useful in the treatment of painful menses and for nervous exhaustion in either sex.

BLUE COHOSH

Another Native American Indian remedy, blue cohosh was originally used to ease the pain of labor. It is believed to relieve uterine spasm and to regulate menstrual flow, particularly to induce a period. Like squaw vine, it also has diuretic properties that may help ameliorate female hormonal fluid accumulation. It is used very effectively with either of the two preceding herbs for these indications. It is also recommended in the treatment of heavy menses. In summary, then, blue cohosh is considered a useful herb for painful uterine spasm related either to menses or menopause and to regulate a disordered menstrual flow.

Herbs Used Topically

*7*he herbs considered in this chapter are frequently used topically (applied directly to the skin) to treat a wide variety of skin conditions. Their enormous popularity gives explicit testimony to their effectiveness. They are among the most commonly employed of all herbal products. Although these herbs have all been used internally, we will concentrate on external application only.

ALOE

Aloe is an immensely popular herbal remedy today, but this should not obscure the fact that its use originated over 2,000 years ago. It has always been highly valued in the treatment of minor cuts and skin irritations and is most effective in the treatment of insect bites—and, most especially, sunburn. It is believed by many to have a "drawing quality" and has been recommended for use in preventing and treating infections of the skin.

Direct application of the gel is particularly soothing, and aloe plants are found in many a sun worshiper's home. A host of creams and lotions containing aloe are also effective and widely available. Aloe is a useful addition to any herbal medicine chest because it provides relief in virtually all minor skin conditions, especially burns.

WITCH HAZEL

Witch hazel can be useful for minor skin irritations and is soothing for minor bruises and cuts. It was first used by North American Indians but today can be found in virtually any home medicine cabinet. Witch hazel can be considered for use in practically all minor skin problems and is highly regarded in the external treatment of varicose veins and hemorrhoids.

COMFREY

Comfrey is used externally as a healing agent. It is employed in a whole host of injuries and lesions that are more serious or substantial than those treated by the agents mentioned above. It has been called "boneset" and has been used by orthopedic surgeons in the treatment of fractures since its constituent active ingredients contract, forming a "plaster."

It also contains allantoin, which is believed to stimulate the formation of new bone, cartilage, and connective tissue. It therefore helps in the repair of skin injuries and has been called "healing herb." It is present in both over-the-counter healing remedies (Unicare Lotion) and prescription medications (Herpecin, Vagimide Cream). Comfrey is best considered an herb used externally for use in more serious or significant skin injuries, where its healing properties are much esteemed.

A Summary of the Herbs and Their Reputed Effects

Aromatic Digestives (Warming)

ANGELICA

Increases appetite

Improves digestion

Used as antispasmodic (gut)

Used for colic

Antigas

Expectorant (drying)

CARDAMOM

Increases appetite

Improves digestion

Used in pregnancy for morning sickness, headache

CINNAMON

Improves digestion

Used as antispasmodic (gut)

Used for colic

Antigas

Controls diarrhea

Used for gastroenteritis

FENNEL

Increases appetite

Used for colic

Relieves intestinal cramps

Antigas

Used for hiccups

Used for gastroenteritis

Stimulates milk production

Bitter Digestives (Cooling)

DANDELION

Improves digestion

Beneficial for gallbladder

Used for gallstones

Beneficial for liver

Used for arthritis (used as diuretic)

Used for kidney problems

Used for urinary tract stones

Helpful for swollen breasts

GENTIAN

Increases appetite

Improves digestion

Used for arthritis

GOLDENSEAL

Soothes mouth irritation (mouthwash)

Soothes throat irritation (gargle)

Soothes vaginal irritation (douche)

Used for esophagitis (inflammation of the esophagus)

Used for gastritis (inflammation of the stomach)

Used for ulcers

MILK THISTLE

Protects liver from injury

Helps liver restore itself

YELLOW DOCK

Used for eczema

Used for psoriasis

Used for arthritis

Helpful laxative

Vasodilators (Warming)

CAYENNE

Induces cleansing sweat

Improves digestion

Used for headache

Used for cluster headache

Used for arthritis

Improves peripheral circulation (blood supply to the extremities)

Increases effectiveness of other herbs in the mixture

FEVERFEW

Used for headache

Used for migraine

Used for arthritis

GARLIC

Builds up defenses against infection

Used as expectorant

Used in respiratory infections

Helpful in asthma

Used for gastroenteritis

Lowers cholesterol

Inhibits blood clotting

Counteracts atherosclerosis

GINGER

Induces cleansing sweat

Used for gastroenteritis

Controls nausea

Controls vomiting

Controls diarrhea

Used as expectorant (drying)

Used in respiratory infections

Improves peripheral circulation (blood supply to the extremities)

GINKGO   *150   21.95*

Improves memory

Improves brain function (cognitive)

Increases cerebral circulation

Improves peripheral circulation (blood supply to the extremities)

Inhibits blood clotting

Used for tinnitis (ringing in ears)

Used in depression

HAWTHORN   *250. 19.95*

Opens coronary arteries

Lowers heart rate

Maintains normal heart rhythm

Lowers cholesterol

Increases strength of heart muscle contractions

Improves peripheral circulation (blood supply to the extremities)

Used for hypertension

Sedatives and Antispasmodics (Cooling)

CHAMOMILE
Used for anxiety

Used for nervousness

Relieves stomach cramps

Used as antispasmodic (gut)

Used for colic

Antigas

Helpful for mastitis (painful breasts)

Helpful for painful periods

Helpful for menopausal symptoms

HOPS
Used for anxiety

Used for restlessness

Used for nervousness

Used for insomnia

Relieves intestinal cramps

Helpful in irritable bowel syndrome

Antigas

Controls diarrhea

PASSIONFLOWER
256 /8.95

Used for anxiety (more severe cases)

Used for nervousness (more severe cases)

Used for insomnia (more severe cases)

Used for tension headache

PEPPERMINT
Used for anxiety

Used for nervousness

Used for insomnia

Used as antispasmodic (gut)

Used for colic

Antigas

Used for gastroenteritis

Controls nausea

Controls vomiting

Used for headache

VALERIAN

Used as a tranquilizer

Used for anxiety

Used for nervousness

Used for insomnia

Used for headache

Used for tension headache

Recommended for childhood behavioral disorders

Diuretics

HORSETAIL

Diuretic (especially for hormonal edema associated with menopause)

Used for arthritis (used as diuretic)

Used for skin problems (used as diuretic)

Increases calcium absorption

Used for hypertension

PARSLEY

Diuretic

Used for arthritis (as diuretic)

Relieves intestinal cramps

Antigas

Used to bring on a period

Helpful for premenstrual syndrome

Used for hypertension

UVA URSI

Diuretic

Used to prevent urinary tract infection

Used to treat urinary tract infection

Used for urinary tract infection (relief of symptoms)

Cold Medications and Expectorants

ELECAMPANE

Expectorant (drying)

Dries excessive respiratory secretions

Antibacterial in lung

Used in gallbladder disease

Used in liver disease

MA HUANG

Dries excessive respiratory secretions

Used in asthma (relieves bronchospasm)

Used for the common cold

Used in flu

Used for hay fever

THYME

Expectorant (moistening)

Loosens respiratory secretions

Antibacterial in lung

Used in asthma (relieves bronchospasm)

WILD BLACK CHERRY

Antitussive (cough suppressant)

WILD CHERRY BARK

Antitussive (cough suppressant)

Cleansing Herbs

BURDOCK

Used in eczema

Used in psoriasis

Used for canker sores

Used for boils

Used for carbuncles

Used for acne

Used for arthritis

Diuretic

DEVIL'S CLAW

Used for arthritis (pain relief)

ECHINACEA   250   24.95

Builds up defenses against infection

Boosts immune function

Used in all infections

Used in eczema

Used in psoriasis

Used for canker sores

Used for boils

Used for carbuncles

Used for acne

Used in cancer

MYRRH

Soothes mouth irritation (mouthwash)

Soothes throat irritation (gargle)

Soothes vaginal irritation (douche)

NETTLE

Used in eczema

Used in psoriasis

Used for canker sores

Used for boils

Used for carbuncles

Used for acne

Used for arthritis

Diuretic

Helpful in diabetes (lowers blood sugar)

Stimulates milk production

Helpful in premenstrual syndrome

Tonic Herbs

GOTU KOLA

250 17.95

Nervous system relaxant

Improves brain function (cognitive)

Increases memory

Used for phlebitis

LICORICE

Establishes emotional balance

Establishes mental balance

Establishes physical balance

Expectorant (moistening)

Used in asthma (relieves bronchospasm)

Used for respiratory infections

Used for gastritis

Used for ulcer

Helpful laxative

Used in arthritis

OATS

Used in depression

Used in melancholia

Nervous system restorative

Nervous system stimulant

Used in neuralgia

Used in shingles

Used in multiple sclerosis

SAINT-JOHN'S-WORT

Used in anxiety

Used for tension

Used for insomnia

Used in depression

Nervous system restorative

Nervous system relaxant

Used for bed-wetting (not due to physical causes)

Helpful in irritable bowel syndrome

Helpful for painful periods

Helpful for menopausal symptoms

Chinese Tonic Herbs

ASTRAGALUS

Increases energy (especially for the physically active)

Builds up defense against infection

Boosts immune function

Used in cancer

DONG QUAI

Increases energy

Regulates menses generally

Used to bring on a period

Helpful for painful periods

Helps regulate irregular or frequent periods

Helpful for menopausal symptoms

Helpful for premenstrual syndrome

Used in pelvic infections

Opens coronary arteries

Maintains normal heart rhythm

Lowers cholesterol

Improves peripheral circulation (blood supply to the extremities)

FENUGREEK

Increases energy (especially in convalescence)

Helpful in diabetes (lowers blood sugar)

Stimulates milk production

Used as an aphrodisiac

GINSENG

Establishes emotional balance

Establishes mental balance

Establishes physical balance

Reduces stress

Increases energy

Antiaging

Used as an aphrodisiac

Male Hormonal Herbs

DAMIANA

(handwritten:)50   17.95)

Used in anxiety

Used in depression

Used for headache

Used as an aphrodisiac

SEVEN BARKS

Antiaging (male)

Diuretic

Used for urinary tract stones

SAW PALMETTO

Antiaging (male)

Increases energy (especially in convalescence)

Used for urinary tract infection

Used for benign enlargement of prostate (BPH)

Used as an aphrodisiac

Female Hormonal Herbs

BLUE COHOSH

Regulates menses generally

Helpful for painful periods (uterine spasm)

Used to bring on a period

Helps regulate irregular periods

Helps regulate frequent periods

Helpful for menopausal symptoms (uterine spasm)

Diuretic

Used for pelvic inflammation

DONG QUAI

(see Chinese Tonic Herbs, p. 78)

SQUAW VINE

Helpful for painful periods

Used to ease childbirth

Diuretic

Used for nervous exhaustion

Herbs Used Topically

ALOE

Used for minor cuts and skin irritations

Especially soothing for sunburn

COMFREY

Used for more serious injuries

Forms a "plaster" used to treat fractures

Stimulates formation of new bone, cartilage, and connective tissue

WITCH HAZEL

Used for minor cuts and bruises

Used for varicose veins and hemorrhoids

PART *3*

In this section we will consider commonly encountered diseases and symptoms and the herbs most useful in their treatment. Chapters are arranged by organ systems for easy access to information. Flowchart diagrams are also included, each proceeding from more general symptoms to more specific. The diagrams keep similar symptoms or indications together in order to facilitate the location of the most suitable herb.

Like most remedies, herbs may not always be effective, and you may decide to call the doctor after an unsuccessful trial of herbal therapy for mild, nonthreatening symptoms. Never feel embarrassed to do so, and always tell the doctor exactly what herbs you have been taking and their effects.

It is important to have your primary care physician aware that you are using herbs. This doctor should be someone with a favorable attitude toward herbal therapy. At a minimum you have the right to expect empathy and open-mindedness. Any physician who is clearly antagonistic toward herbalism may well be equally narrow-minded about other controversial issues, and such dogmatism has no place in a healer. Physicians are entitled and indeed obligated to educate, but they should not dictate.

As stated in the cautionary note at the beginning of this book, herbs should never be considered as a substitute for professional consultation and care. If you are ill, first call a well-trained and tolerant physician; if in doubt, always err on the side of prudence and call. Never, never say, "Let's try these herbs first and see whether they help." Herbal medicines should be employed only after you have decided that the doctor is not needed.

However, remember that you do not need to visit the doctor for each minor ache and pain, and most minor illnesses require symptomatic treatment at most. The common cold will run its course in two weeks if you see an M.D. and fourteen days if you do not. Thus an increase in self-reliance in matters of health may be quite positive.

For example, physicians are commonly seen for mild sore throats and ear pain, minor coughs, and swollen glands. In many such cases, the cause of these ills is viral. Although antibiotics are both necessary for and curative of bacterial infections (such as strep throat), they are of no use in viral illnesses.

However, having consulted the doctor, the patient anticipates that an antibiotic will be given, and often the physician will acquiesce. After all, if he fails to do so, the patient will leave the office dissatisfied, may complain to friends and family members, and will probably see another doctor who will write the desired prescription. So rather than trying to educate the patient, he fulfills his expected role, prescribes an antibiotic, and everyone is pleased.

While there is certainly no malicious intent, this practice has two negative consequences. First, indiscriminate use of antibiotics contributes to the emergence of resistant bacteria—strains that do not respond to treatment with conventional antibiotic therapy and can cause life-threatening infections.

The second effect, while more insidious, is equally pernicious. It fosters an unnecessary dependence on the doctor and organized health care as the only source of cure and healing. It encourages us to accept a passive role in matters of health and discourages questioning those with positions of authority in the health care hierarchy.

I genuinely believe that these are unintentional effects of a health care system that have evolved over the past hundred years, and that the vast majority of physicians have only their patients' best interests at heart. But I affirm with equal sincerity that we must begin to take a more active part in the maintenance of our own health, be informed participants in our own care, and be less dependent on others for our continuing wellness. As you become more acquainted and comfortable with herbal healing, you will assuredly gain great satisfaction and enjoyment from being an active participant in ensuring your own health.

Cardiovascular Disease

etermining the significance of troubling symptoms always requires expert professional advice. *If you have any suspicion that you may have any form of heart disease, a qualified practitioner must be consulted. Self-treatment in this area is reckless and potentially life-threatening.* However, with your physician's awareness, herbal remedies may well be employed in cardiovascular disease, either alone or with prescribed medications. They are also used as preventive measures in those prone to heart disease, and especially for those who want to take an active role in maintaining their good health.

In the area of prevention, herbal remedies should not be considered a substitute for a healthy lifestyle. Not smoking, consuming a diet low in saturated fat and cholesterol, regular aerobic exercise, and maintenance of ideal body weight are known to maximize cardiac health. A tranquil, peaceful demeanor, a feeling of contentment with the world, and harmony in your relationships are also believed to be antidotes to coronary disease. While not a complete list, these form the basis for any plan of cardiac wellness.

The first heart problem we will consider is coronary heart disease (see Figure 1.) The usual manifestations are chest pain related to exertion (angina), or sudden severe chest pain that may be associated with nausea, vomiting, sweating, or shortness of breath (signs of a possible heart attack). Here the basic problem is a narrowing of the arteries (atherosclerosis) that feed blood and oxygen to the heart muscle. Short of prevention, the most direct approach to this problem is to open the affected arteries (see Figure 1, #1.)

Of all the herbal remedies, hawthorn is probably most specifically employed for this effect. Indeed, hawthorn is, in my opinion, the most useful herb used in the treatment of heart disease. It has been shown to lower blood pressure, help protect against atherosclerosis, and improve circulation to the heart. Dong quai has also been recommended as a coronary vasodilator.

Garlic is reputed to have an antiatherosclerotic effect (see Figure 1, #2.) Along with ginkgo, it is believed to inhibit the clotting of blood (considered the immediate cause of heart attack) and to lower cholesterol levels. Thus it is useful both in the prevention and treatment of coronary disease—all with no unwanted side effects. Both hawthorn and dong quai are reputed to lower cholesterol levels as well.

Normally the heart beats regularly (rhythmically, without syncopation) and at a set frequency (usually about seventy-two times a minute). Irregular (syncopated) or unusually slow or rapid heart rates are termed arrhythmias. Both hawthorn and dong quai are believed to normalize heart rhythm (see Figure 1, #3). Hawthorn is also used when lowering the heart rate may be beneficial, as in some cases of angina.

While some arrhythmias are benign, others may be life-threatening, and a careful analysis of their significance by a qualified physician is mandatory. Because modern drugs used to treat arrhythmias are plagued with frequent and potentially serious side effects, they should be used only when absolutely indicated.

Hypertension (high blood pressure) requires professional help for diagnosis, treatment, and appropriate follow-up (see Figure 1, #4.) The options for treatment are varied, and an open discussion of the alternatives should be encouraged. Physicians have learned that the medications employed to treat high blood pressure are not innocuous, so some may recommend a nonpharmacological approach to control.

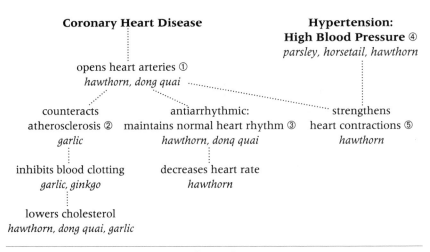

Coronary Heart Disease

Hypertension:
High Blood Pressure ④
parsley, horsetail, hawthorn

opens heart arteries ①
hawthorn, dong quai

counteracts
atherosclerosis ②
garlic

antiarrhythmic:
maintains normal heart rhythm ③
hawthorn, donq quai

strengthens
heart contractions ⑤
hawthorn

inhibits blood clotting
garlic, ginkgo

decreases heart rate
hawthorn

lowers cholesterol
hawthorn, dong quai, garlic

FIGURE 1

Specifically, in overweight patients weight loss may be all that is needed to lower elevated blood pressure. Moderating intake of salt or excessive alcohol may be sufficient to stabilize blood pressure in other patients. An intermediate step before utilizing prescription antihypertensives may be the use of herbal remedies. Herbal diuretics, especially parsley and horsetail, have been utilized to lower blood pressure, and hawthorn has been purported to help also.

Congestive heart failure can result from either coronary heart disease or hypertensive heart disease. In fact, symptoms of heart failure represent a final common expression of inadequate cardiac function and can develop in any form of heart disease (congenital, rheumatic, and so on). The most common manifestations are shortness of breath, usually associated with exertion or on lying flat, or swelling of the ankles. Hawthorn is said to benefit the heart muscle, increasing the strength of each contraction, and thus may be used in cases of congestive heart failure (see Figure 1, #5.)

Circulatory Problems

A general feeling of coldness, particularly in the extremities, may be the manifestation of a functional decrease in blood flow. Herbs with a general stimulating effect on the overall circulation, like cayenne and ginger, may be beneficial in such cases (see Figure 2, #1).

Problems of arterial circulation to the extremities (see Figure 2, #2) may benefit from graded exercise, smoking cessation, and prescription drugs when warranted. Hawthorn, dong quai, and ginkgo are also said to open up the arteries and may be advantageous in peripheral arterial disease.

Gotu kola is used in the treatment of thrombophlebitis (inflammation of the veins, most common in the calves). It is said to reduce swelling and pain (see Figure 2, #3). Numerous studies have shown gotu kola to be beneficial in a wide range of venous problems.

Ginkgo is considered advantageous in most common venous problems as well. Like gotu kola, it has been utilized in cases of phlebitis and it is also of reputed benefit in the treatment of varicose veins (see Figure 2, #3).

Risking redundancy, I would like to underscore the need for professional help in diagnosing and treating the conditions considered in this chapter. With that understanding, it is my opinion that the use of herbs to treat heart problems will increase dramatically in the next decade.

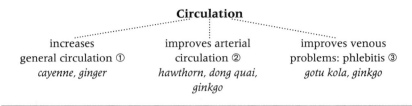

Circulation

increases general circulation ①	improves arterial circulation ②	improves venous problems: phlebitis ③
cayenne, ginger	*hawthorn, dong quai, ginkgo*	*gotu kola, ginkgo*

FIGURE 2

Some of the most widely prescribed cardiac drugs have come under close scrutiny over the past two decades, and their side effects have been documented to be far more widespread and serious than anticipated. As a result, the use of diuretics to treat high blood pressure and antiarrhythmics to treat irregular heartbeats has been drastically curtailed. Herbal therapies, largely free of untoward effects, will be increasingly utilized as continuing research documents their effectiveness and physicians become more open to alternative therapies.

Respiratory Disease

*C*ough is a primary symptom of disease of the respiratory system (Figure 3, #1). Cough lasting more than a week or associated with fever may indicate a serious condition and should be evaluated by a physician. Cough is most often caused by infection of the respiratory tract, allergies, or direct physical irritation (for example, cigarette smoke). With this in mind, it is easy to understand the concept of encouraging the cough reflex. The removal of the cause of distress is considered the basis of any therapeutic regimen in traditional herbal medicine. Expelling the insulting pollen, the irritating soot, or the disease-causing organism makes good sense.

The body has an innate tendency toward self-healing, and the first goal of any therapeutic system is to encourage and maximize that urge. This explains the contrast between herbalists, whose cornerstone respiratory medicinal is the expectorant to encourage cough, and the modern pharmacy replete with cough suppressants.

In contemporary terms, cough is generally described as productive or dry. A productive cough is characterized by excessive amounts of phlegm. The drying expectorants help dry out excessive mucous secretions and stimulate their removal. Ginger, elecampane, garlic, angelica, and ma huang (see Figure 3, #3) are all commonly used herbs in this class.

The efficacy of these drugs is believed to be enhanced by the concomitant use of a diuretic, such as parsley. This combination of diuretic and drying expectorant is believed most efficient in drying up and mobilizing excessive bronchial secretions.

When the cough is dry, the moistening expectorants are favored (see Figure 3, #4). Thyme is the classic herb in this class and is said to loosen up or decrease the stickiness of respiratory secretions and encourage their elimination. (Licorice has similar properties and may be considered in this class although it contains some components with drying properties as well; therefore when a significant humidifying effect is desired, thyme is the better choice.)

Asthma is characterized by excessive responsiveness of the airways to any irritative influence, resulting in spasm of the air passages (see Figure 3, #2). Asthmatic attacks can result from allergies, infection, pollutants, emotional factors, and even weather changes. In the susceptible individual, the net effect of any of these provocative factors is spasm of the bronchial tree, which is experienced by the patient as difficulty in breathing.

Herbs have a long history of effective use in the treatment of asthma. Thyme is said to relax airway spasm, so it is recommended for the asthmatic with a dry cough. In fact, because it is almost always desirable to produce a moistening effect on an asthmatic's airways, thyme is an ideal herb in virtually all cases.

Licorice is found by many to be a most useful herb in asthma. It is said to increase the production of cortisone, which relieves airway spasm, and to act generally as a moistening expectorant. In those rare cases when a drying expectorant is required in an asthmatic, garlic and ma huang may be used with good effect. However, it should be repeated that a moistening effect is nearly always indicated in these cases.

All the drugs mentioned are believed to be effective in the treatment of respiratory tract infections (see Figure 3, #6). Garlic is a particularly valued herb for treating lung infections. It is excreted via exhalation and exerts a disinfecting effect on the lung. Thyme is also highly regarded and is believed to have a disinfecting or cleansing effect. Elecampane is also thought to be active against disease-causing

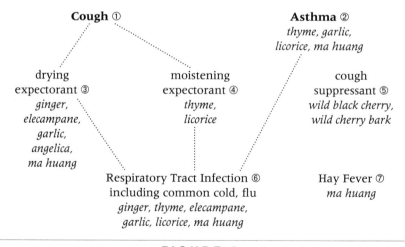

Cough ①

Asthma ②
thyme, garlic, licorice, ma huang

drying expectorant ③
ginger, elecampane, garlic, angelica, ma huang

moistening expectorant ④
thyme, licorice

cough suppressant ⑤
wild black cherry, wild cherry bark

Respiratory Tract Infection ⑥
including common cold, flu
ginger, thyme, elecampane, garlic, licorice, ma huang

Hay Fever ⑦
ma huang

FIGURE 3

organisms. Ginger and licorice are also reportedly beneficial in the treatment of respiratory infections. However, if infection is suspected (fever, yellow or green sputum), a physician should be consulted since, in addition to one of the above, an antibiotic may be warranted.

Ma huang is an extremely useful herb in treating the most common respiratory ailments. By effecting a relaxation of the airways and a drying of secretions it aids in the expectoration of sputum. It is frequently employed in the treatment of the common cold or flu. It is also of great benefit in allergic respiratory problems like asthma (mentioned above) and hay fever. An active ingredient derived from this plant forms the basis of popular over-the-counter cold remedies, but those who have utilized the whole herb attest to its greater effectiveness. Its multiple effects are highlighted in Figure 3.

The last herbs to be considered are the antitussives wild black cherry and wild cherry bark (see Figure 3, #5). These drugs are used only when cough is debilitating, countertherapeutic, or superfluous (for example, a nervous cough or a cough preventing a restful night's sleep). However, in herbal medicine this group of drugs is infrequently indicated, since elimination of the offending agent is part of the herbal credo. And, most importantly, one does not attempt to thwart the body in its business of self-healing.

Diseases of the Urinary Tract

*I*n both scientific and alternative medical systems, the diuretics are the most widely used drugs that affect the urinary system. Western medicine uses these agents in two commonly encountered clinical situations: high blood pressure and fluid retention states. Thus diuretics are among the most commonly employed of prescription medications.

Within the herbal tradition, however, there are even further indications for these drugs. The elimination of waste material, resulting from normal metabolic processes in the body or taken in from the environment, has long been an herbal prerogative. As mentioned earlier, the herbalist sees the accumulation of toxins as being commonplace in disease states and always seeks to enhance the body's natural bent to evacuate these poisons.

Most herbal mixtures will have some effect on elimination. In many toxic or inflammatory conditions, the preferred route of removal is the urinary tract. In particular, skin problems that appear inflammatory (associated with redness or heat) or are of long duration, as well as joint problems, are believed to benefit from an herbal diuretic. Thus they are employed in the treatment of many common skin problems (eczema, psoriasis, canker sores, boils, carbuncles, and acne) and in the full range of arthritic conditions. Diuretics, in short, are used in Western medicine (e.g. for high blood pressure) and they are used in alternative medicine (for arthritis and skin problems). In both scientific and herbal medicine, diuretics are used to treat fluid retention.

A word about safety. Most prescription diuretics cause a loss of potassium in the urine, thus depleting the body's potassium level. This is a major concern in their long-term use. Most plant material, including herbs, is naturally high in potassium, so that loss of potassium is rarely a problem.

All the herbs listed as diuretics (see Figure 4, #1) aid in the elimination of fluid and waste from the body. All may be used, therefore, in states of fluid accumulation or in a treatment program for high blood pressure. Their further characterization may aid in choosing a diuretic in individual cases, however. For example, seven barks is subclassed as a diuretic favored for men (see Figure 4, #2). The reason for this relates to other known properties of seven barks, other characteristics which recommend its use for men.

In addition to its diuretic properties, it is specifically believed to have an antiaging effect in men. Therefore in a middle-aged male with high blood pressure, seven barks might be an obvious choice. Similarly, a woman may well benefit from the use of squaw vine or blue cohosh (see Figure 4, #3) when a diuretic is indicated, because of other advantageous effects these herbs have on women. Horsetail is specifically indicated for hormonal edema (swelling) related to the menstrual cycle or menopause.

The cleansing diuretics are believed to have a particular effect on the elimination of toxins. They are commonly employed in inflammatory skin conditions and arthritic conditions that are believed to benefit from this approach (see Figure 4, #4). There is no scientific documentation and no clear-cut evidence that these maladies are indeed caused by an accumulation of "poisons." The use of these herbs in such cases is based, rather, on a long history of clinical experience; these illnesses are seen to benefit from the use of these remedies. Such empirical evidence has often been relied on as a foundation for treatment long before a scientific explanation is discovered, even in Western medicine. Why should it not be equally acceptable in an herbal framework?

Horsetail is widely favored as the diuretic most useful in inflammatory skin conditions. Along with parsley and dandelion, it is commonly employed as a cleansing diuretic in arthritic conditions. Their use will be discussed in appropriate chapters.

Overall, the most favored herb in the treatment of infections of the urinary tract is uva ursi (see Figure 5, #1). It is believed to be an effective urinary tract antiseptic and is useful both in the prevention

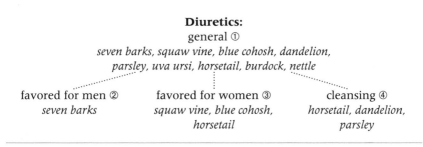

Diuretics:
general ①
seven barks, squaw vine, blue cohosh, dandelion,
parsley, uva ursi, horsetail, burdock, nettle

favored for men ②	favored for women ③	cleansing ④
seven barks	*squaw vine, blue cohosh, horsetail*	*horsetail, dandelion, parsley*

FIGURE 4

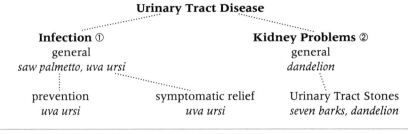

FIGURE 5

and treatment of urinary tract infections. In addition, it is believed to have a soothing effect on the urinary tract and is utilized to help relieve the troublesome symptoms of urinary tract infections (burning, pain). However, it is important to consult a physician if you suspect a urinary tract infection because antibiotics may be required for treatment.

Saw palmetto is also considered to be useful in the treatment of urinary tract infections generally. It is particularly indicated, however, when there is concomitant enlargement of the prostate gland (a common cause of such infection in older men) for which it is said to be beneficial. (See Chapter 16.)

Dandelion is one of the most venerated of herbal remedies. As such, it has transcended its reputation as a diuretic and is, in some herbal traditions, believed to be useful in the treatment of kidney problems generally (see Figure 5, #2). Among these problems is urinary tract stones, a condition that seven barks is also believed to benefit. However, urinary tract stones or any disease involving the kidney itself warrants a medical consultation before any therapeutic approach is initiated.

I believe that the herbs in this chapter offer interesting insights into the herbal approach to health. For example, the herbal diuretics can be recommended for use in the treatment of hypertension or fluid retention. However, the herbalist senses an additional usefulness in these drugs over and above the mundane.

The notion of a medicine as somehow benefiting the overall, global functioning of an organ (as dandelion for the kidney), or acting to rid the body of impurities (as in the cleansing diuretics) may strike us as somewhat quaint or archaic. But it is notions like these that many of us find most enticing and challenging about herbal medicine. Indeed, many a Western physician would attest that the effects of his efforts often surpass those predicted by pure science.

CHAPTER 23

Gastrointestinal Disorders

*T*his chapter illustrates a decisive difference between alternative and modern Western medicine. It may be something of an oversimplification, but scientific medicine generally views its patient as either ill or well. Conversely, the herbalist sees a gradation from illness to wellness. The function of many herbs may best be defined not so much as curative but rather as enhancing wellness. In other words, one need not actually be ill to benefit from herbal therapy.

Herbalists generally believe that some degree of debility or predisposition to illness will generally precede the development of the illness itself. If one is at less than maximal wellness, the opportunity exists to utilize certain herbs in order to achieve full vitality and thus become less susceptible to disease.

Our modern pace of life, with tremendous stress and pressure; inadequate exercise, recreation, and rest; overly processed and hastily consumed food; and lack of time for peaceful reflection leaves us all in a less than optimal state of health. Many herbalists would see none of us as especially healthy. They would say we all could benefit from herbal treatment.

Similarly, if one is ill, the notion of increasing one's physical resources and increasing one's strength in order to facilitate recuperation would be considered equally valid by an herbalist. All of this should sound familiar; it is but another example of the basic herbal dogma of helping the body to heal itself, maximizing the body's ability to execute its self-healing privilege.

The first group of herbs we will consider in this chapter bears directly on this concept. I have labeled their attribute "Nutritional Enhancements," and Figure 6 shows a further division into two subfunctions: increasing appetite and increasing digestion.

In scientific and alternative medicine, but most especially in alternative medicine, much of the body's vitality and energy is believed to be derived from the food that we eat (see earlier discussion of *qi* in

Nutritional Enhancements

increases appetite
cardamom, angelica,
fennel, gentian

improves digestion
cardamom, cinnamon,
angelica, cayenne,
gentian, dandelion

FIGURE 6

Chapter 4). The herbalist sees an increase in the ingestion (eating), digestion (absorption), and assimilation (incorporation into the body) of foodstuffs as a paramount focus. It is the most direct method available to strengthen the body that is at less than peak level and the surest way to facilitate a complete recuperation.

Virtually everyone today would benefit from an improvement in nutritional status and thus vitality. Therefore, many herbal mixtures contain a foundation herb either from the aromatic or bitter digestive categories. Any of the herbs in these groups favorably influences absorption and assimilation of foods and could serve as a base herb in a mixture.

For a patient who is sluggish or fatigued or who appears to require a degree of stimulation, one would choose from the warming herbs of the group (cardamom, angelica, fennel, cinnamon, cayenne). Both cardamom and angelica would be considered excellent choices here, with cardamom especially favored for those who are chronically ill. In the much more commonly encountered situation today where a cooling, relaxing herb is indicated, gentian would seldom be wrong. As both an appetite stimulant and digestive aid it is without peer.

Parenthetically, I would briefly mention here that horsetail (see Figure 7) is thought to increase absorption of calcium. Fenugreek and nettle (see Figure 7) are believed to lower blood sugar in diabetics, thus having a positive effect nutritionally. However, if you suspect diabetes, it is important to consult a physician.

Lowers Blood Sugar
fenugreek, nettle

Increases Calcium Absorption
horsetail

FIGURE 7

We will now consider the use of herbs to treat specific maladies of the gastrointestinal tract. After a brief discussion of liver and gallbladder disease, the most frequently experienced symptoms of dysfunction of the stomach and intestines and their herbal remedies will be presented.

In herbal tradition, the health of the gallbladder and that of the liver are interconnected. Herbs that benefit the gallbladder are often seen to be advantageous for the liver as well. Both dandelion and elecampane are believed to stimulate bile production and to provide overall benefit to the gallbladder and liver. By diluting the bile, dandelion is said to benefit the patient with gallstones (see Figure 8, #4). If gallstones are suspected I recommend medical consultation before beginning any therapeutic regimen.

The price that we pay for the affluence and plenty of contemporary life is a constant barrage of potentially dangerous chemicals both in the food we eat and the air we breathe. Additives, preservatives, insecticides, toxic waste, many types of pollutants, and nuclear debris are all new to this century. The liver, as the organ charged with the responsibility of metabolizing and detoxifying these chemicals, is under great strain. Add to that our occasional proclivities to excessive ingestion of known liver toxins (drugs, nicotine, alcohol) and the burden can become overwhelming. Thus hepatics, or liver tonics, are highly prized in contemporary herbal medicine (see Figure 8, #2 and 3).

Milk thistle is currently in great favor in Europe as a hepatic. It is believed both to protect the liver from injury and to aid in the liver's regenerative attempts after injury. It therefore may be useful in the recovery phases of hepatitis.

Inflammation of the upper gastrointestinal tract is due to irritation of the digestive tube by acid produced in the stomach. Esophagitis, gastritis, or ulcer (if more severe) are the medical terms used to denote such conditions. In lay parlance, we refer to indigestion, dyspepsia, heartburn, or sour stomach.

Two herbs have been found to be most beneficial in alleviating these symptoms (see Figure 9). Goldenseal has long been considered an extremely soothing and healing herb when applied to the mucous membranes (lining cells of the body cavities) and is considered

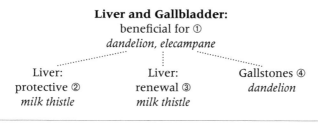

Liver and Gallbladder:
beneficial for ①
dandelion, elecampane

Liver:	Liver:	Gallstones ④
protective ②	renewal ③	*dandelion*
milk thistle	*milk thistle*	

FIGURE 8

Upper Gastrointestinal Inflammation

Esophagitis	Gastritis	Ulcer
goldenseal	*goldenseal, licorice*	*goldenseal, licorice*

FIGURE 9

particularly useful for inflammatory conditions of the upper gastrointestinal tract. Licorice is also a very useful herb in these conditions. It provides symptomatic relief, perhaps by stimulation of a protective mucous, and is believed to encourage healing in cases of ulcer disease.

Although both these herbs can be highly recommended for these indications, symptoms of any duration or associated with any bleeding should be brought to a physician's attention.

Disordered contraction of the muscles lining the digestive tract causes spasm of these muscles, which is experienced as a gripping pain in the abdomen that can be quite severe. It can be due to a myriad of causes. Many of these are quite benign and include flulike illnesses, food allergy, mild cases of food poisoning, or even anxiety. In some cases, no cause can be determined. Occasionally, however, spasm may be the result of an intraabdominal catastrophe requiring immediate medical attention. This possibility must always be considered when there is associated fever, severe pain, or tenderness.

Cinnamon, angelica, chamomile, and peppermint are generally employed antispasmodics. (See Figure 10, #1.) All are believed to decrease hyperactivity in the gut and relax the abnormal contractions of the intestinal musculature. All have been effectively employed to this end. If, in addition, a calming or relaxing effect is desired (that is, if anxiety, tension, or nervousness is believed to be contributing to the development of spasm) one would favor the use of chamomile or peppermint.

Chamomile has developed a particular reputation for use in cases of "nervous stomach" (see Figure 10, #2). Here its properties as an antispasmodic and gentle relaxant are most effectively utilized and provide significant comfort and relief. For cramping pain developing lower down in the digestive tract, you should consider fennel, parsley, or hops. All are found to be effective, but hops probably have developed the greatest renown in the treatment of intestinal cramping because their trait as a relaxer of muscle tension is believed to be most centered in this area. As a sedative and calming herb, hops are particularly recommended for use in irritable bowel syndrome (see Figure 10, #3 and 4). Saint-John's-wort has also been used in this disease.

All of the general antispasmodics (see Figure 10, #5) have been employed in the treatment of colic, but fennel has possibly the longest and most widely acclaimed history of use for this disorder and seems to be particularly effective in infants.

Gastrointestinal Spasm:
general ①
cinnamon, angelica, chamomile, peppermint

Cramps:	Cramps:	Colic: ⑤
stomach ②	intestine ③	*cinnamon, angelica,*
chamomile	*fennel, parsley, hops*	*fennel, chamomile,*
		peppermint

Irritable Bowel Syndrome ④
hops, Saint-John's-wort

FIGURE 10

Gastroenteritis, most commonly due to a viral infection of the digestive tract, is in most cases an unpleasant but short-lived malady. Symptomatic treatment is in order and begins with restricting one's oral intake initially to clear liquids. Bland foods (toast, cooked cereal) may be added as symptoms abate. Herbs used in the treatment of gastroenteritis have included cinnamon, fennel, ginger, peppermint, and garlic (see Figure 11, #1). The herb or herbs employed will depend on the primary symptoms being experienced. Ginger and peppermint (see Figure 11, #2 and 3) have often been favored when nausea predominates and are thus the favored herbs to prevent vomiting as well. (Ginger is also often utilized in morning sickness during pregnancy.)

Cinnamon, ginger, and hops have all been effectively utilized in controlling the diarrhea that frequently complicates the clinical picture (see Figure 11, #4). Cinnamon has long been a favorite remedy

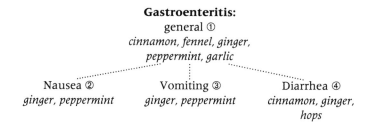

Gastroenteritis:
general ①
cinnamon, fennel, ginger,
peppermint, garlic

Nausea ②	Vomiting ③	Diarrhea ④
ginger, peppermint	*ginger, peppermint*	*cinnamon, ginger,*
		hops

FIGURE 11

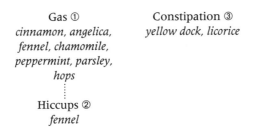

Gas ①
*cinnamon, angelica,
fennel, chamomile,
peppermint, parsley,
hops*

Constipation ③
yellow dock, licorice

Hiccups ②
fennel

FIGURE 12

for mild gastrointestinal infections. If spasm or gripping pain is also present, hops might well be considered for use. I must also give garlic its due and note that its advocates would consider it a first-choice drug in any case of gastroenteritis, particularly since it is said to have a sterilizing effect on disease-causing organisms in the gut.

In their general tonifying effects on the digestive tract, many of the aromatic and bitter digestives are found to be effective at dispelling gas (see Figure 12, #1 and 2). Therefore, if one is treating any of the problems discussed earlier in this chapter and gas is a concurrent problem, it is likely that the remedy employed will also allay excessive gaseousness. Specifically, cinnamon, angelica, fennel, chamomile, peppermint, parsley, and hops have all been effectively utilized in this regard. Fennel may be particularly effective when hiccups are present.

Both yellow dock and licorice have been used as herbal laxatives. Yellow dock has been used since ancient times, and licorice finds favor in use with children (see Figure 12, #3). Senna, which acts by adding bulk to the stool, is also commonly employed.

This concludes our consideration of herbs used for their effects on the gastrointestinal tract. I have tried to demonstrate the herbalist point of view that the gut is not only the target of disease but can also be utilized in the considerably more positive role of promoting wellness.

The herbalist hopes that the digestive herbs will be utilized not just to relieve symptoms of acute illness, but to enhance the nutritional state and increase overall vigor and vitality. This can play an important role in a program to ensure enduring wellness.

CHAPTER 24

Arthritis

*A*rthritis is a catch-all term signifying that there is inflammation of a joint. Such inflammation commonly causes swelling and pain of the affected area, and these symptoms are among the most frequent prompting a physician's evaluation.

Causes of arthritis are legion. The most common form of arthritis (osteoarthritis) is believed to be due to wear and tear on the joints as a result of weight bearing, injury, or other mechanical stresses. Some cases of arthritis are due to abnormal deposits of crystals within joints (gout); others are associated with acute infections (arthritis associated with gonorrhea).

Arthritis may be a manifestation of disease in another area of the body—for example, arthritis associated with bowel problems or psoriasis. A particularly crippling form of arthritis (rheumatoid arthritis) can ultimately affect other organ systems. This list is far from complete, but is simply meant to demonstrate that arthritis is a common symptom with a multitude of causes. In some cases of arthritis, a good deal is known about the mechanisms involved in joint inflammation; in others there is only speculation. If joints swell, stiffen, or become inflamed, it is best to see a doctor because these symptoms may indicate serious medical conditions.

A host of prescription drugs are available to aid in the treatment of arthritis. When this situation exists one can immediately make two assumptions. The first is that the disease is common; the horde of pharmaceutical companies would not be working on new drugs for a particular ailment unless it affected a lot of people. (Finding a cure for a common disease is much more profitable than curing an uncommon disease.) Second—and this is a good general rule of thumb—whenever the pharmacy stocks an entire aisle of drugs to treat a problem, none is particularly effective over another. Obviously if one drug is decidedly better than the others, the less advantageous drugs disappear from use. Drugs that are clearly superior will rapidly replace less efficacious ones. In the case of arthritis, many are indeed quite helpful for some patients, but clearly no panacea has been found, and they are all fraught with potentially hazardous side effects.

The great safety of herbal therapies offers a major advantage here. This is of particular significance because, in most cases, arthritis is a chronic illness and will require lifelong medication, at least intermittently if not continuously. And a last point before getting to the herbs themselves: any case of arthritis of acute or sudden onset, especially if associated with redness or swelling, or any case not responding to herbal treatment, warrants a physician's evaluation and treatment.

Gentian (see Figure 13, #1) has been used for gout (an acute and particularly painful form of arthritis) and is believed to have properties that neutralize the painful inflammatory response so characteristic of the disease. It is now considered a useful herb in all forms of arthritis.

Cayenne, as a circulatory stimulant, increases the blood flow and is believed to aid in the body's healing efforts. It has a long history of topical use in herbal therapeutics, being utilized as a poultice or compress in arthritic cases. A "new" cream for such use with capsicum (derived from cayenne) as its active ingredient has recently been marketed. Oral preparations are also effective.

Regardless of the route of administration, the goal is the same: increase the circulation and supplement the body's natural restorative processes as opposed to simply relieving troublesome symptoms. Feverfew also has been used in arthritic cases, generally with much the same rationale as cayenne. They are both believed to have anti-inflammatory effects, but this should be interpreted in the sense of decreasing the painful elements of inflammation.

Since both are circulatory stimulants, they should be considered as supporting the positive aspects of inflammation (the body healing itself). Licorice, believed to stimulate the body's production of cortisone, is a time-honored treatment for the pain and inflammation of arthritis. It is but another example of the herbalist's imperative of allowing the body to help itself. Rather than giving the patient cortisone, the herbalist prefers to give a natural herb that will stimulate the body to make more of that which it needs. It underscores a basic respect for nature and the desire to meddle as little as possible.

To the herbalist, most cases of arthritis are believed to benefit from cleansing away an accumulation of harmful material. Some forms of human arthritis fit well with this herbal model of toxins or

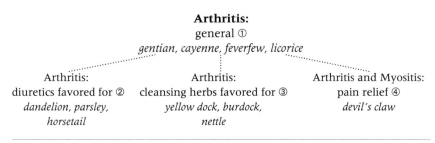

Arthritis:
general ①
gentian, cayenne, feverfew, licorice

Arthritis:	Arthritis:	Arthritis and Myositis:
diuretics favored for ②	cleansing herbs favored for ③	pain relief ④
dandelion, parsley, horsetail	*yellow dock, burdock, nettle*	*devil's claw*

FIGURE 13

accumulation, while others clearly do not. The use of diuretics (see Figure 13, #2) and cleansing herbs (see Figure 13, #3), however, should not be viewed on this theoretical level. They are used, first and foremost, because they have gained a reputation for being useful or helpful in the management of arthritic conditions.

The herbalist is much less interested in the mechanism of *how* something works than in *whether* something works. Consequently, the diuretics dandelion, parsley, and horsetail and the cleansing herbs yellow dock, burdock, and nettle have developed a particular renown for being useful in the arthritic diseases. This is based on a great deal of clinical experience shared among herbalists and not on experiments done in test tubes in a lab. While both have their place, the herbalist prefers the former.

Devil's claw (see Figure 13, #4) may be particularly useful as an analgesic (pain reliever) in the treatment of arthritis. As such, it often improves mobility and use of the affected joint, which further enhances healing. It is also used for muscle pain and inflammation (myositis).

A general approach to arthritic problems might well begin with a combination of a purifying herb (diuretic or cleansing herb) along with one of the more broadly efficacious arthritic remedies (see Figure 13, #1). Some degree of trial and error may be necessary to find the most effective blend in each case. When pain and immobility are severe, devil's claw may be added. Severe cases of arthritis also warrant evaluation by a physician.

Neurological Disorders

O f all disorders affecting the nervous system, the most mundane but also the most common cause of distress is headache. Headache is such a universal malady that few people can say they have never experienced one. The vast majority of headaches are benign. However, the following warning is in order: any change in the frequency or severity of headaches should prompt a medical evaluation. It may signal a more serious underlying problem.

Many herbs have been employed in the symptomatic treatment of headache. Damiana, cayenne, feverfew, valerian, and peppermint all have a history of widespread and successful use for headache in general (see Figure 14, #1).

Certain herbs are believed to be especially helpful in specific headache syndromes. Migraine headaches (throbbing in nature and often associated with nausea and vomiting) are believed to be particularly responsive to feverfew (see Figure 14, #2). Studies have found it to be effective when taken to prevent migraine, and it is also effective in aborting an attack already in progress.

Cluster headache, a particularly severe variant that can occur nightly for weeks, is believed to benefit from the use of cayenne (see Figure 14, #3). In tension headache, where anxiety or nervousness often plays a role, it is not surprising that the sedative herbs valerian and passionflower are useful (see Figure 14, #4).

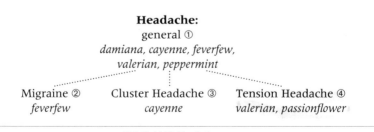

Headache:
general ①
damiana, cayenne, feverfew,
valerian, peppermint

Migraine ②   Cluster Headache ③   Tension Headache ④
feverfew   *cayenne*   *valerian, passionflower*

FIGURE 14

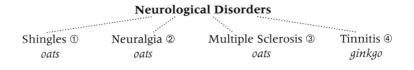

Neurological Disorders

Shingles ①	Neuralgia ②	Multiple Sclerosis ③	Tinnitis ④
oats	*oats*	*oats*	*ginkgo*

FIGURE 15

Oats have been used in a variety of neurological disorders in-cluding shingles, neuralgia, and multiple sclerosis (see Figure 15, # 1, 2, and 3). Self-diagnosis and treatment of these conditions is not suggested or recommended.

Tinnitis, or ringing in the ears, in some cases may benefit from treatment with ginkgo (see Figure 15, #4).

One's general state of vigilance or level of arousal can also be in-fluenced by herbs. Certain of these are found to act as nervous sys-tem stimulants, while others act as relaxants. I am using the terms "stimulant" and "relaxant" as a measure of alertness or preparedness as opposed to indifference or unconcern. Oats (see Figure 16, #1) tend to make one more aware and watchful and are therefore con-sidered to be a central nervous system stimulant. On the other hand, Saint-John's-wort and gotu kola (see Figure 16, #2) are believed to have a relaxing effect on the nervous system, lowering one's level of excitability.

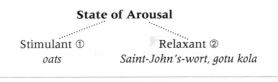

State of Arousal

Stimulant ①	Relaxant ②
oats	*Saint-John's-wort, gotu kola*

FIGURE 16

Gotu kola, which was just cited as a nervous system relaxant, has been used for fully two thousand years as an Asian remedy. But it is only of late that it has become popular in the West, and it is now developing a reputation here for enhancing intellectual functioning (see Figure 17). It is believed to function particularly as a memory aid and to facilitate problem-solving ability (cognitive function). Whether this is due to its relaxant effect on the brain, an increase in cerebral circulation, or some unknown mechanism is undetermined at this time, but the herb's proponents are vocal in their support.

Ginkgo (see Figure 17) has been shown to advance mental acuity and improve memory in young and old alike. This is largely attributed

Intellectual Functioning

improves memory
gotu kola, ginkgo

improves cognitive function:
clarifies thought processes
gotu kola, ginkgo

FIGURE 17

to its effect on cerebral circulation, but a direct effect on the nervous system is also postulated.

While this chapter began with the very ordinary subject of headache, I will conclude with more lofty notions like mental balance and nervous system tonic. Such ideas seem somewhat archaic in our scientifically rigid times, where experiments and numbers seem to possess more validity than concepts or ideas. Yet the belief that a group of herbs can have a positive effect on the overall functioning of an organ or body system has a strong basis in alternative medicine.

Oats and Saint-John's-wort (see Figure 18, #1) are believed to enhance, renew, and revive the nervous system. They are seen as having an invigorating effect, increasing energy and stamina. In cases of debilitation, particularly after an exhausting illness, they are believed to rejuvenate the nervous system and restore it to its state before illness. They are considered to be supportive and nourishing, and to replenish or replace what has been lost.

Ginseng and licorice (see Figure 18, #2) are believed to contribute to a sense of balance on the mental level. They will augment a quality when it is lacking, and they will decrease it when there is an excess. If the scales are unequal they will add to one side or subtract from the other, whichever is indicated, until stability is achieved. They ease the tension between opposing mental states (such as calm versus agitated, contemplative versus frivolous) and restore the mind to a state of equilibrium and peace.

Nervous System Tonics

nervous system restoratives ①
oats, Saint-John's-wort

improves mental balance ②
ginseng, licorice

FIGURE 18

Psychiatric Disorders

*L*ike the herbs in the preceding chapter, those we will discuss here have their primary effect on the nervous system. Many of these herbs were discussed in Chapter 25 with respect to their effects on neurological disorders. In that chapter, we concentrated on the physical or more concrete plane. In this chapter, we will discuss the action these and additional herbs have on psychiatric disorders. Thus, we will now consider effects that predominantly influence the mood or feeling of the individual. In cases of serious emotional disturbance, you are well advised to consult a qualified psychologist or psychiatrist, or some other health care professional who can refer you to one.

The first group of herbs we will consider is calming and is therefore used to counteract a state of anxiety both generally and in its more specific manifestations. Damiana, valerian, passionflower, chamomile, peppermint, hops, and Saint-John's-wort have all been utilized to allay the sense of uneasiness or apprehension that we associate with anxiety (see Figure 19, #1). They are all believed useful in general anxiety states, but some particular tendencies make certain of these herbs more useful in individual situations.

Damiana, in addition to relieving anxiety, seems to promote a general feeling of contentment. Valerian is particularly effective when there is headache associated with anxiety, and passionflower is also utilized in this setting (see Chapter 25). Passionflower, in addition, has often been favored in the more severe cases of anxiety.

Chamomile has been used for thousands of years for anxiety and is especially recommended when symptoms of a nervous stomach predominate. Peppermint also is commonly utilized when anxiety is associated with stomachache or queasiness. When intestinal cramps and spasms are the primary manifestations of anxiety, hops are the favored herb. Saint-John's-wort is particularly recommended when there is a degree of agitation or hyperexcitability.

Valerian (see Figure 19, #2) is a respected herbal tranquilizer considered by many to be as effective as prescription drugs but without having a sedative effect or potentiating the effects of alcohol. Valerian, passionflower, chamomile, peppermint, and hops (see Figure 19, #3) have all functioned to relieve the agitation and uneasiness associated with nervousness.

Aside from considerations mentioned earlier, there is little to favor one over another in this application except that, true to its general reputation, passionflower seems to be more effective in more severe cases. Hops (see Figure 19, #4) appear to be effective in cases of restlessness. The strain associated with nervous tension is believed to respond most effectively to the use of Saint-John's-wort (see Figure 19, #5).

Insomnia is a common problem, almost symptomatic of our highly pressured lives and our seeming inability to escape the coercive demands being made on our time. Our brains seem always to be on fast forward, and we are unable to slow them down even in our attempts to fall asleep. Here again, herbs can be of benefit. But, not surprisingly, some simple, fundamental lifestyle changes may also provide a fitting basis for lasting benefits in all these anxiety-related conditions. In the Chinese system of wellness, balance is of fundamental importance. Thus, rest and exercise would represent two fundamental balancing tendencies. In such a scheme a regular planned period of daily exercise would be believed to contribute to a peaceful, restful sleep.

Similarly, the constant pressures of work, societal, and family demands could well be balanced by a period of quiet reflection, meditation, or prayer. The often antagonistic or at least adversarial interplay that can occur between employer and employee and in numerous other encounters during the day can be balanced by a supportive and sharing conversation with a friend. These basic but essential changes could take one a long way in relieving the common symptoms we are describing in this chapter.

Valerian, passionflower, peppermint, hops, and Saint-John's-wort (see Figure 19, #6) are all said to be effective in securing a good night's sleep. Saint-John's-wort, which is considered a nervous system restorative, may provide more long-lasting benefit, as described in Chapter 25, while passionflower is considered effective in more severe cases. Saint-John's-wort (see Figure 19, #7) is believed to benefit children who suffer from enuresis (bed-wetting) when the cause is not physical.

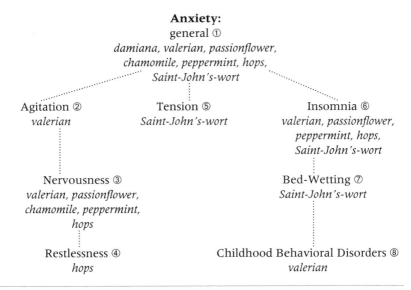

Anxiety:
general ①
damiana, valerian, passionflower,
chamomile, peppermint, hops,
Saint-John's-wort

Agitation ②   Tension ⑤   Insomnia ⑥
valerian   *Saint-John's-wort*   *valerian, passionflower,*
peppermint, hops,
Saint-John's-wort

Nervousness ③   Bed-Wetting ⑦
valerian, passionflower,   *Saint-John's-wort*
chamomile, peppermint,
hops

Restlessness ④   Childhood Behavioral Disorders ⑧
hops   *valerian*

FIGURE 19

Childhood behavioral disorders, especially learning disabilities and hyperactivity, have responded to the use of valerian (see Figure 19, #8). In a large study involving 120 children, a host of behavioral parameters were evaluated. Seventy-five percent of the youngsters given valerian showed improvement in symptoms including restlessness, bed-wetting, nail-biting, and learning and behavioral disorders. Of great clinical importance was the lack of unwanted side effects.

Damiana, oats, Saint-John's-wort, and ginkgo (see Figure 20) have all been seen to provide benefit in the depressive disorders, and oats are believed to be beneficial in more severe cases of melancholia as well. Saint-John's-wort may be preferred in cases of agitated depression, when a hyperexcitable state coexists with depression. Remember that severe anxiety, depression, or hyperexcitability warrants evaluation by a professional.

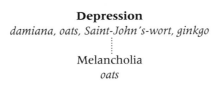

Depression
damiana, oats, Saint-John's-wort, ginkgo

Melancholia
oats

FIGURE 20

Emotional Balance
ginseng, licorice

Stress Reduction
ginseng

FIGURE 21

Ginseng is believed to be useful in the specific area of stress reduction. But in a broader sense, ginseng and licorice are both believed to encourage a state of balance in the emotional milieu (see Figure 21). This is quite analogous to a similar function played by these herbs in the neurological realm. Thus they can be seen as supplying what is lacking or taking away that which is in excess. Their role is to move the individual to the middle ground emotionally.

On the neurological level, they were seen as easing the tension existing between opposing mental states; I used the examples of calm versus agitated and contemplative versus frivolous. On the emotional level, ginseng and licorice would be seen more as balancing aspects like courage versus fear, optimism versus pessimism, or joy versus sadness.

This may sound odd to the Western mind, but one must remember the importance herbalists ascribe to balance. Excesses, even of qualities like joy (generally considered beneficial), are considered deleterious. Likewise, emotions like fear or sadness, discouraged in the Western mentality, are considered essential in Eastern thought.

Those who appreciate music or art understand that a musical composition demands a soft passage in order to build to a fitting crescendo, and a painting requires darkness for the light to really glow. In Eastern philosophy the same is true with feelings or emotions; all must be experienced and a harmony must be maintained. This is the foundation of true peace.

CHAPTER 27

Virility and Male Reproductive Disorders

*T*he herbs in this chapter are all cited elsewhere in this book, where their applications in treating a variety of ailments that can affect both males and females are discussed. Therefore, these herbs can be used with good effects in both sexes. They each, however, have particular applicability in the treatment of uniquely male problems, and it is on these actions that this chapter concentrates.

I have, somewhat tongue in cheek, labeled seven barks and saw palmetto as virility herbs consonant with the chapter's title (see Figure 22, #1). To be more accurate, these herbs are said to prevent or forestall the negative consequences of aging in the male, thus contributing to a continuance of virility into old age. Seven barks and saw palmetto are discussed at greater length in Chapter 16.

Several herbs are said to have aphrodisiac qualities (see Figure 22, #2 and 3). Not surprisingly, these are among the most commonly used of herbal medicines. Ginseng and fenugreek are "equal opportunity" aphrodisiacs believed to be similarly effective in renewing sexual interest in both men and women.

Although saw palmetto is seen as possibly effective in both sexes, it is believed to be perhaps more beneficial in the male. Damiana is said to be helpful to both sexes when psychological difficulties are thought to be contributing to flagging sexual activity. It is believed to enhance sexual execution as well, particularly in the male.

Saw palmetto is believed useful for symptomatic treatment of noncancerous enlargement of the prostate in aging men (see Figure 22, #4). Important note: I recommend medical consultation in all cases of difficulty urinating or any sign of blood in the urinary stream, common signs of prostate problems in males. Likewise, difficulties of sexual function of any duration merit professional evaluation.

Virility Herbs ①
seven barks, saw palmetto

Aphrodisiac ②
*ginseng, fenugreek,
saw palmetto*

Benign Prostate Hypertrophy ④
saw palmetto

Aphrodisiac:
psychological ③
damiana

FIGURE 22

Female Reproductive Disorders

*A*bnormalities of the normal female monthly reproductive cycle are unfortunately common and cause a great deal of anxiety and suffering in the women affected. Fortunately, these problems do not usually indicate serious underlying pathology. However, any symptoms that cause concern should be brought to a physician's attention. Regular gynecological checkups are of course recommended.

A group of herbs found to be particularly effective in menstrual disorders will be considered in this chapter. As mentioned in the discussion of male reproductive herbs, these medicines also have more general applications and can be used without reservation in both sexes, but we will concentrate on their strictly feminine usages here.

The herbs used in an attempt to regulate the monthly cycle and ease the discomfort associated with menses in the broadest sense are dong quai and blue cohosh. I will give them the general accolade of menstrual cycle normalizer (see Figure 23, #1). Since a regular cycle depends upon a precise balancing of hormones over a specific time sequence, we can envision these herbs as contributing to this balance and thus stimulating hormone release on some occasions and inhibiting release on other occasions. I don't mean to indicate that there is any understanding of whether or how this is accomplished. Rather it is a way of visualizing what is happening conceptually, which is similar to our perceptions about other herbs (for example, licorice and ginseng). The important thing is that these herbs have a lengthy reputation for reestablishing a normal menstrual flow where this was previously lacking.

In addition to a general normalizing effect on the monthly cycle, certain herbs have developed a particular reputation for use in more specific functional aberrations. Dong quai and blue cohosh are both utilized to bring on a suppressed menstrual flow; blue cohosh is particularly advocated in this role. Parsley has also been used successfully (see Figure 23, #2).

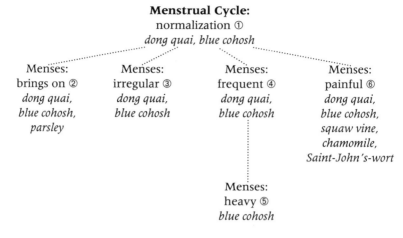

Menstrual Cycle:
normalization ①
dong quai, blue cohosh

| Menses:
brings on ②
dong quai,
blue cohosh,
parsley | Menses:
irregular ③
dong quai,
blue cohosh | Menses:
frequent ④
dong quai,
blue cohosh | Menses:
painful ⑥
dong quai,
blue cohosh,
squaw vine,
chamomile,
Saint-John's-wort |

Menses:
heavy ⑤
blue cohosh

Premenstrual Syndrome ⑦
dong quai, horsetail, parsley, nettle

Menopause ⑧
dong quai, blue cohosh,
Saint-John's-wort, chamomile,
horsetail

FIGURE 23

Dong quai and blue cohosh likewise have been applied to irregular and frequent menses and have been found to have a normalizing effect. Blue cohosh has also been used to check a heavy menstrual flow (see Figure 23, # 3, 4, and 5).

Painful menses (dysmenorrhea) is an important problem sometimes causing great discomfort. Dong quai, blue cohosh, squaw vine, chamomile, and Saint-John's-wort (see Figure 23, #6) are all believed effective in relieving this problem. However, when uterine spasm seems to be the predominant distress, squaw vine and blue cohosh are believed to be the most salutary. Chamomile offers an antispasmodic property that is thought to relieve gynecological symptoms. It affords a gentle relaxing effect that may be a bonus in some cases. Likewise, in addition to its muscle-relaxing qualities, Saint-John's-wort can be helpful when anxiety or emotional tension add to the monthly distress.

Dong quai, parsley, and nettle have all been used effectively in the treatment of premenstrual syndrome (see Figure 23, #7). Since hormonal abnormalities have been implicated in the genesis of premenstrual syndrome, especially if there is disordered menstrual function, normalization of menstrual flow with the herbs mentioned above should go a long way to relieving premenstrual distress. Since fluid retention is often a cardinal feature of the syndrome, horsetail may also be a useful adjuvant. Finally, any associated nervousness, anxiety, or depression should be addressed as needed.

For menopausal symptoms (see Figure 23, #8) one also has a choice of effective herbs. Dong quai has long held an estimable reputation for symptomatic relief of uncomfortable menopausal symptoms (hot flashes, sweats). Blue cohosh is said to be particularly effective when uterine spasm is especially troublesome. Saint-John's-wort, as mentioned with respect to painful periods, is particularly useful when there is an element of anxiety or emotional tension. The relaxing effect of chamomile may also be useful in treating menopause. Horsetail appears to be especially useful in controlling hormonal edema associated with this syndrome.

The controversial issue of estrogen replacement therapy for menopause is beyond the scope of this book. Advocates are vocal in their support while opponents are rightfully concerned about the safety and potential side effects of long-term hormone usage. For readers deliberating this important question, I recommend reading an unbiased book (both sides should be fairly presented) and having an honest discussion with a physician who knows your health history and that of your family.

As I mentioned in Chapter 27, ginseng and fenugreek are considered aphrodisiacs equally effective when used by women or men (see Figure 24). Saw palmetto, while used in both sexes, is perhaps considered more likely to be of benefit in the male. Damiana is believed to be effective for decreased libido in both sexes when there is a considerable psychological component.

Aphrodisiac
ginseng, fenugreek, saw palmetto

Aphrodisiac:
psychological
damiana

FIGURE 24

Cardamom is an aromatic digestive with a long history of use in pregnancy. It has been found helpful in alleviating many of the discomforts associated with pregnancy but seems to provide greatest relief for the associated headache and morning sickness (see Figure 25, #1.) Squaw vine (see Figure 25, #2) has been used by North American Indians to facilitate labor and rapid delivery. Its use should first be discussed with the involved health care professional. If agreed upon, it

Pregnancy:
symptoms ①
cardamom

Childbirth:
easing ②
squaw vine

FIGURE 25

should be initiated several weeks before delivery for maximum effectiveness. Herbs, like all medications, should be used at the lowest possible dose and for the shortest possible duration during pregnancy.

The pain of pelvic inflammation is believed to respond to blue cohosh, and pelvic infections have been said to respond to dong quai (see Figure 26). Medical consultation is indicated in these conditions prior to the initiation of any herbal regimen.

Pelvic Inflammation
blue cohosh

Pelvic Infection
dong quai

FIGURE 26

Dandelion has been said to reduce the swelling of engorged breast tissue, and chamomile has been advocated to relieve pain in mastitis (see Figure 27, #1 and 2). When a woman is breast-feeding, fenugreek, fennel, and nettle are all believed to support the breasts in their providing milk (see Figure 27, #3).

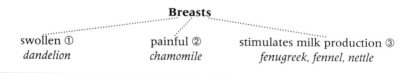

Breasts

| swollen ① | painful ② | stimulates milk production ③ |
| *dandelion* | *chamomile* | *fenugreek, fennel, nettle* |

FIGURE 27

This concludes our survey of herbs used to treat specifically female problems. They have a long history of use (some for millennia) and have been found to be effective when appropriately employed. However, it is worth repeating that none should be considered a substitute for regular medical checkups, including Pap tests and mammography. Troubling symptoms should always be investigated without delay.

Physical Imbalance and Exhaustion

*O*ne could examine the *Physicians' Desk Reference* one page at a time, investigate the scientific medical literature in its entirety, and nowhere find prescription drugs comparable to the herbs we will discuss in this chapter. The functions that these herbs are believed to perform, and the accomplishments with which they have been credited, have no equal in Western scientific medicine.

Western drug classifications are straightforward, scientific, and easily understood. Narcotics relieve pain, antibiotics kill bacteria, decongestants allow for easier breathing, enzymes aid digestion, and so on. The herbs considered in this chapter are said to have qualities that elude such simple categorization. The notion of herbs that can be utilized to increase energy or promote a state of physical balance seems somehow transcendent or metaphysical. The idea that herbs can have an antiaging effect encourages one to set sail again in search of the fountain of youth. Yet these are but some of the qualities ascribed to the tonic herbs.

In our cynical and pessimistic era, such conceptions are easily cast aside as capricious and whimsical. And although we would guard against taking any such claims too literally, we feel that a little magic, taken in small doses and with a hefty chaser of reality, never did anyone any harm.

The first of the tonic herbs we will consider are ginseng and licorice. We have encountered these herbs previously in Chapters 25 through 28 (on neurological, psychiatric, and male and female reproductive herbs). In this chapter we will go beyond these concrete effects to a more intangible realm. Here they are believed to promote an overall sense of equilibrium or stability (see Figure 28).

If one were to take the two physical extremes of, for example, lethargy and hyperactivity, these herbs are said to move one from either extreme to a more appropriate balance point in the middle

Physical Balance
ginseng, licorice

Nervous Exhaustion
squaw vine

FIGURE 28

ground. One could proceed a step further and postulate that these herbs will indeed encourage the appropriate state at the appropriate time.

Herbalists believe that good health requires a balancing of opposites: hard work or exercise must be offset by an appropriate degree of rest. If an imbalance exists in the cycle of rest and activity, these herbs may act to invigorate the individual, enabling the required physical training. On the other hand, when rest is required, they may encourage a peaceful sleep.

A similar effect could be proposed for other physical extremes—for example, constriction versus dilation, absorption versus excretion, contraction versus relaxation—but it should be stressed that the mechanism whereby this is accomplished is by no means understood.

Squaw vine (see Figure 28) is considered rejuvenative in states of nervous exhaustion. Ginseng (see Figure 29) is believed to have properties that stave off the effects of aging. It is obviously not considered an herb that grants eternal youth, or we'd have a large population of 5,000-year-old Asians. Rather, it is believed to foster a youthful vitality of thought and action, and to endow one with the physical vigor to perform accordingly.

Seven barks and saw palmetto (see Figure 29) are believed to forestall the ravaging effects of aging but specifically in the male. The feeling engendered about these herbs is that seven barks and saw palmetto are in some sense protective against the debilitating effects of old age (senility, loss of physical strength) while ginseng is a more active principal infusing qualities which we associate with youth (enthusiasm, potency, curiosity).

Antiaging
ginseng

Antiaging:
male
seven barks, saw palmetto

FIGURE 29

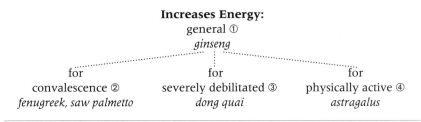

FIGURE 30

Not surprisingly for an herb said to possess antiaging attributes, ginseng is also believed to increase energy (see Figure 30, #1). Studies done in several countries have corroborated this clinical impression, and thus the invigorating effects of ginseng are well substantiated.

Several herbs have also gained a reputation in this area but in more specific settings. In patients who are recuperating from illness, fenugreek and saw palmetto (see Figure 30, #2) are both believed to be advantageous. They are considered to increase strength and quickly restore a full measure of vitality. In cases of severe illness, dong quai is used in the period of convalescence (see Figure 30, #3). Its reputation, particularly in Asian medicine, is in being able to restore those who have had serious and especially debilitating diseases. Long-term use is often recommended. Astragalus is believed to be an energizing remedy and is particularly preferred by those who are physically active (see Figure 30, #4).

The herbs described in this chapter are said to favorably influence some of the most basic qualities of human life (enthusiasm, harmony, vitality) and protect us against the great adversary: aging. Ginseng, a prototype drug in this class is, accordingly, perhaps the single most widely used and prized of all herbal medicines.

Those who choose to use the herbs represented in this chapter must do so, however, with realistic goals. Expecting to run a four-minute mile, become an indefatigable lover, master theoretical physics, or undo the effects of seven decades of neglect will result only in disappointment and frustration. For better or worse, miracles need to be rare events.

However, to repeat a phrase used earlier in this chapter, a "little magic" may be easier to come by. If we are content with more modest benefits, tune in to our body, and listen to its messages, we may find ourselves more favored than we might rightfully expect.

CHAPTER 30

Skin Problems

*H*erbalists believe that people with skin problems benefit from the use of eliminative herbs. Thus herbal prescriptions for dermatologic problems will often begin with an attempt to augment the removal of toxins or poisons. The use of a diuretic would be a particularly popular choice today, and horsetail (see Figure 31, #2) is considered most effective for use in skin problems. Therefore, we could reasonably begin our prescription with horsetail, which is used primarily as a diuretic (see Figure 31, #2).

Yellow dock, burdock, nettle, and echinacea are frequently used for common skin problems (see Figure 31, #1). These have been found to be helpful in cases of eczema and psoriasis. Burdock, nettle, and echinacea have been used with good results in the treatment of canker sores. In addition, the more characteristically infectious skin problems (boils, carbuncles, and acne) are also believed sensitive to the same three herbs (see Figure 31, #3).

In referring back to Part Two of this book, you will find this trio of cleansing herbs discussed in Chapter 13. In addition, yellow dock, although broadly classed as a bitter digestive, is also believed to have significant blood cleansing properties. It is interesting that horsetail,

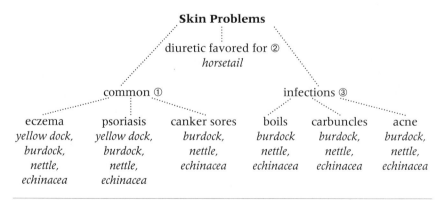

FIGURE 31

Mucous Membrane Irritation

mouth irritation	throat irritation	vaginal irritation
goldenseal, myrrh	*goldenseal, myrrh*	*goldenseal, myrrh*

FIGURE 32

a powerful diuretic, is also believed to have significant cleansing properties that augment its diuretic effect.

Thus, what might evolve as a quite reasonable herbal prescription for most common skin problems would be a combination of a diuretic with a strong reputation for excretion of accumulated toxins (horsetail) with an effective cleansing herb (for example burdock, nettle, or echinacea). While I am not generally in favor of such a "cookbook" approach, many skin problems could be treated advantageously with such a formula.

Goldenseal and myrrh (see Figure 32) have been advocated for use in cases of mucous membrane irritation and may be used for irritation of the mouth (as a mouthwash), throat (as a gargle), or vagina (as a douche).

Naturally, any skin condition not found responsive to the above measures and any suspicious pigmented lesion should be brought promptly to a physician's attention.

CHAPTER 31

Infections

*T*his chapter will deal with the problem of infectious diseases in a general sense. I will not attempt to deal with specific infectious agents or sites of infection but rather will discuss some general herbal principles that are widely applicable to infectious illnesses. It must be stated at the onset that these concepts apply only to mild, self-limited, low-grade infections. Most such diseases are caused by viruses, and antibiotics are of no value in such cases. In any instance where a more serious infirmity is suspected, medical attention should be sought. While I do not wish to understate the value of herbal ministrations in the treatment of infections historically, we now have effective antibiotics, and these must be accorded primacy when indicated.

The induction of a cleansing sweat is largely limited to the folklore of herbalism. It can be considered as part of the general herbal tendency toward elimination as a therapeutic goal. The notion was to raise the body temperature and enhance excretion of the pathogenic influence via the sweat glands.

While the picture of the sweat lodge with burning coals is relegated to antiquity, the concept of provoking a mild warming or sweat by oral administration of ginger or cayenne (see Figure 33, #4) is still favored by some. Its advocates believe that it may be most advantageous in the difficult chronic lingering infections, where such an effort at dislodgment may be just what is needed to give the body the upper hand in the battle.

Echinacea has, in modern times, developed a singular reputation for use in infectious diseases. It is recommended, in a general sense, by virtue of its proposed ability to help in localizing (and thus preventing the spread of) infection. It is also said to have antiseptic and antiviral properties (see Figure 33, #1).

Echinacea is also believed to augment the ability of white blood cells to fight infection, thus enhancing bodily defenses. Garlic and astragalus are also believed to fortify the body's resistance to infection

Infections: **Produces Cleansing Sweat** ④
general ①   *ginger, cayenne*
echinacea

defends against ②   boosts immune function ③
astragalus, garlic, echinacea   *astragalus, echinacea*

FIGURE 33

(see Figure 33, #2). Both echinacea and astragalus are believed to boost immune function (see Figure 33, #3), thereby increasing the body's defensive fortification.

Infections of specific organ systems (for example lung, gut, or urinary tract) are discussed in the appropriate chapters. There are those who would advocate the use of echinacea in virtually all infections and would include it in regimens for infections at these sites as well.

Again, antibiotics should never be neglected when indicated. If in any doubt, seek your doctor's opinion.

PART 4

In this, the last and most comprehensive part of the book, I will try to put together all that has been presented so far. In addition to formulating your individual herbal prescription, I will review the basic notions of alternative healing and thought, and I will incorporate them into recommendations for a lifestyle that makes as much good sense today as it did millennia ago when first proposed. Finally, I will combine principles from scientific, herbal, and alternative medical thinking in a complementary approach to HIV and cancer.

Your Personal Herbal Prescription

*T*his is the most ambitious and rewarding chapter in the book. It is also the most important chapter because it represents a benchmark in your taking greater responsibility for your own well-being and maximizing your own good health.

In this chapter, the effort you have put into thoughtfully reading this book will be repaid. You are now prepared to formulate your own herbal mixture, a preparation as individual as you are, and that addresses your temperament and your needs at this moment in time. This is your wellness prescription. It is meant for daily use so that you can enjoy life to the fullest with maximal radiant good health.

During times of infirmity this prescription may need to be altered to augment the body's healing tendencies. Specific information on herbal treatment of common illnesses can be found in Part Three of this book, where symptoms common to each of the major organ systems of the body are considered and appropriate herbs are recommended. The flowchart diagrams, which proceed from general to more specific symptoms, should lead you to the most efficacious herbs for your particular problem. In this chapter, however, we are dealing with an herbal formula that you will use during times of good health.

While the notion of taking medication when you are feeling well is not widely accepted in scientific medicine, it has a strong theoretical basis in more ancient medical settings. Often the scientific physician views health simply as the absence of disease. Herbalists view health as a continuum. While the impotent, dull couch potato and the vigorous, engaging bon vivant may both be described as healthy (that is, free from disease), there is certainly a great disparity in their degree of wellness. The herbalist feels that by the proper prescription of invigorating plants, you can move toward your point of maximal wellness. My goal in this chapter is to assist you in formulating your own personal herbal prescription.

To this end, we will use sound, time-tested principles, and our mixtures will be based on an honest assessment of your own special needs and distinctive personality. With care and thought you will develop an herbal tonic that will help you achieve emotional harmony as well as increase physical vitality. The prescription that evolves will be truly unique, truly yours.

It is perhaps revealing that herbalism relies most often on combinations of herbs rather than "singles." This is in contradistinction to Western medicine where, in general, specific ailments (such as pneumonia) are treated with specific medications (such as penicillin). A clue may be provided by the herbal mindset, in which each person is seen as a composite of physical, mental, emotional, and spiritual selves. These are not seen as distinct or separate but instead are totally merged into an individual whole. Any attempt to help dispel disease or amplify wellness will more likely be successful if multiple levels of the self can be benefited. One thus employs herbs that can act in the physical, mental, and emotional realms. (Spirituality, which in alternative thought includes notions like friendship, art, beauty, and love, is not specifically affected by medicines but rather by one's entire lifestyle, and that is the subject of the following chapter.)

It is of interest that the other great alternative system of healing, acupuncture, likewise involves the use of multiple sites rather than the insertion of a single needle. The typical acupuncture prescription includes placement of needles at several locations in order to achieve the best balance and flow of energy in each individual case. Combination therapy, with simultaneous employment of both herbs and acupuncture, is also commonplace in ancient Asian medicine. Again, this serves to underline the composite nature of man and reminds us that wellness can be best achieved by judicious treatment at all levels.

Today, we tend to think that holistic medicine is a twentieth-century revelation. Rather, ancient forms of healing have, from the beginning, respected and administered to all components that make up each unique person. The depth and intensity of this commitment is echoed in the use both of multiple herbs and of multiple acupuncture points in the quest for healing, as well as the combined use of both modalities in the same patient.

Several guidelines will greatly aid in your developing an appropriate and advantageous prescription. First and foremost is honesty. View yourself as you are, not as you wish you were. Be honest about your faults, shortcomings, and defects. The more carefully you define the person you are now, blemishes and all, the more likely you will be to formulate an herbal prescription to help you become the person you want to be. This is important not only on the physical level but also in your consideration of your emotions and personality. The better you define the problem, the more effective the solution.

Second, limit your prescription to three or four herbs. My personal bias would be to begin by selecting one of the digestive herbs (an aromatic or bitter digestive) and an herb from the tonic or hormonal groups (tonic herbs, Chinese tonic herbs, male and female hormonal herbs). If your temperament is overly placid or dispassionate, a vasodilator would be warranted. At the other extreme, those who are subject to anxiety and excitability would benefit from a sedative or antispasmodic.

One could perhaps add an herb for specific, chronic, recurring, or anticipated medical problems, such as uva ursi for those prone to repeated urinary tract infections, or garlic in those with a strong family history of heart disease. Each of these categories will be considered at length in the remainder of this chapter, along with the rationale for selecting one herb over another.

I would like to emphasize that this approach is my own personal one, and it is not meant to be representative of any consensus of herbal opinion. Instead it is based on an understanding and respect for herbal tradition and herbal pharmacology, and it fits well with accepted notions prevalent in scientific medical thinking.

Choosing a Digestive Herb

Utilizing a digestive herb as the foundation of an herbal prescription makes good sense in both alternative and modern scientific medical frameworks. In ancient Chinese medicine, nutrition is considered a major source of energy, or *qi*. Scientific medicine confirms that we ultimately derive our energy from the foods we eat. This energy is used up, according to both viewpoints, and needs to be replenished every day. Thus, beginning with an herb that is believed to foster more efficient digestion and assimilation of food energy provides a strong basis for any herbal regimen. The digestivë herbs have a beneficial effect on all aspects of digestion. They are believed to increase the appetite, facilitate normal movement of food in the gut, and aid in digestion. The overall result is an increase in available nourishment and an increase in energy.

The digestive herbs are often subdivided into two groups, the aromatic digestives and the bitter digestives. The aromatic digestives, by virtue of their warming nature, are indicated for use by those who tend toward lassitude and apathy. These herbs are also favored in the treatment of most illnesses. As part of a wellness prescription today, the bitters are generally favored. In addition to their positive effects in digestion, the bitters have a calming or pacifying quality that nicely counteracts the modern mentality. Since anxiety, tension, and pressure seem to afflict the majority of twentieth-century Americans, these cooling herbs are more in tune with our needs than the aromatics.

Gentian is a classic bitter herb and is an excellent choice as a foundation herb. It stimulates the appetite and is a superior digestive aid. Its long history of use and unsurpassed safety particularly recommend it for long-term usage. Milk thistle, because of its beneficial effects on the liver, would be a better choice for those who have a history of drug abuse or intemperate use of alcohol. It should certainly be considered by those with a history of hepatitis. Similarly, since many chemicals are broken down in the liver, those especially concerned about pollution or exposure to industrial toxins might consider this herb as their digestive aid. Dandelion is believed to be quite beneficial for those with gallbladder disease and should be considered by patients so afflicted.

Yellow dock is the bitter I would recommend for those with chronic skin or arthritic problems since it is believed to act as an herbal cleanser and is considered beneficial for these conditions. Patients with inflammatory problems of the gut should consider goldenseal as their cornerstone bitter because of its beneficial effects on mucous membranes—the lining cells of the digestive tract, which are affected in ulcer disease, hiatal hernia, gastritis, colitis, and so on. These, then, are the bitters that could well be utilized as a foundation for a wellness prescription.

The aromatic digestives are favored for use in times of debility or poor health. Angelica might be considered primarily for acute conditions, while cardamom is an excellent choice for those with chronic illness. The aromatics are particularly useful in combating specific gastrointestinal symptoms, and thus they tend to be employed most commonly for sporadic short-term use. The typical twentieth-century American—harried, pressured, and deadline-driven—will benefit most from a bitter digestive, and I recommend your choosing from that group except in those circumstances noted above.

Since your wellness prescription will be taken daily, the digestive herb you employ should be taken in the lower dosage range. The subject of dosage is considered in Chapter 5, but an important point needs to be made here. In the context of this chapter we are utilizing the aromatics and bitters as digestive aids, not in an attempt to treat symptoms. Thus, if an herb is recommended at a dosage of, for example, 5 to 15 drops one to three times a day, the higher dosage range (say, 15 drops two or three times a day) may be necessary in the treatment of colic, ulcer, or gallbladder disease. However, for purposes intended here, a dosage of 5 drops two or three times a day is more appropriate. Likewise it is important to recognize that the development of any untoward effects will call for a decrease in dosage or even switching to another digestive herb. As mentioned elsewhere, always err on the side of being overly cautious and conservative. If an herb is well tolerated, the dosage can always be increased if greater effect is desired.

We have, by the simple utilization of one herb, already made positive improvements on two different levels. The aromatics and bitters all augment digestive processes, resulting ultimately in an increase in available energy and enhancement on the physical level. In addition, their qualities as warming (aromatic) or cooling (bitter) herbs will have some effect on the emotional level, energizing those with a lethargic temperament while calming those who tend to be more hyper.

Choosing a Sedative Herb

We live in an era plagued by incessant activity and a permanent state of exaggerated alertness. It is as if we are in high gear at all times, afraid to miss a trick and always guarding against our neighbor's gaining an upper hand. This requires a constant state of vigilance, and the emotional toll is considerable. Like a rubber band stretched to the limit, we live our lives at the breaking point. Many physicians and psychologists feel that this is a major cause of the current epidemic of coronary heart disease. Unquestionably, today's hectic pace contributes mightily to psychological problems, addictive disorders, and many familial and social problems.

Its greatest devastation, though, while less dramatic, is more pervasive and insidious. We go through life stalking like caged animals, our very muscles and sinews taut and ready to pounce. We are fearful and unable to trust; we view everyone with suspicion. While this picture may be somewhat overstated, I feel that this outlook best characterizes the prevailing mood of our time. We live life at the limits, with a vague sense of apprehension and always prepared for the worst. I see a definite relationship between our excited, nervous temperaments and our tendency to view our fellow human beings as potential adversaries rather than as brothers and sisters.

If we could just slow down, calm down and relax, I think we might find ourselves unwittingly bidding each other "good morning," letting each other into our lane on the highway, and maybe even smiling at strangers. We might begin to smell the roses; we might really see the splendor of a brilliant sunset, hear the magic in a robin's song, and experience the wonder, awe, and beauty of being alive.

Achieving this state of mind requires conscious effort and the development of a new outlook. Seeing the world as benevolent and our neighbor as ally and friend takes effort. It is part of a wellness lifestyle, which will be explored in the next chapter. But most of us today must first quiet our agitated, excited, and overactive constitution before even attempting such a transformation.

This is the advantage of employing a sedative herb in your wellness prescription. The sedatives and antispasmodics are the ideal antidote to our frantic times. They have a calming effect, helping to assuage anxiety and promote relaxation, all without any potential for abuse or addiction.

Valerian would be a good basic choice in this category. It is a natural tranquilizer par excellence, and since it is nonsedating, it has no effect on mental acuity or physical prowess. Passionflower similarly is a very effective tranquilizer but should be used only in more severe cases of disquietude since it can cause drowsiness. It is best recommended for short-term use during especially stressful periods.

Chamomile and hops are also useful herbs in this category. Because of their antispasmodic properties they are quite effectively employed by those with an uneasy or sensitive gut. In common usage, hops are favored for irritable colon and associated lower abdominal cramps, gas, and diarrhea, while chamomile is favored for a nervous stomach. Peppermint shares in the relaxant and antispasmodic properties of these herbs and can also be effectively employed.

In my private practice and in my clinic work, virtually all my herbal prescriptions include one of the herbs from the sedative-antispasmodic group. Whether the immediate problem is heart disease, arthritis, hepatitis, or AIDS, a sense of calm and peace can only benefit the overall process of healing.

These herbs are not a cure for all that ails humankind. Rather, they should be seen as a worthwhile first step in a long journey. It is a journey that will require time for solitude; time devoted to the appreciation of art, music, and literature; and even time for meditation and prayer. It will result ultimately in a feeling of comfort with oneself and one's neighbors and a sense of belonging in a benevolent, bounteous world.

If you find yourself unable to muster any significant emotional response to life, if one day seems to merge into the next without any differentiation, if you feel unenthused and apathetic, you should be evaluated for an underlying physical problem or early depression. In my years of practice, I have found that such lassitude almost invariably is symptomatic of an underlying problem and once that difficulty is addressed, a new enthusiasm and joie de vivre become manifest. For the rare person in good health who seems to require an emotional boost, cayenne is considered to have a stimulating effect.

We have now utilized two herbs and have made appropriate adjustments in two spheres. We have improved digestive processes and thus favorably influenced our level of energy. Additionally we are utilizing herbs to bring us to a healthier state emotionally. This is important in itself and prerequisite to the spiritual growth discussed in the next chapter.

Choosing a Tonic or Hormonal Herb

It would be quite reasonable at this point to add one of the tonic or hormonal herbs to your wellness prescription. Ginseng would be an excellent choice for men. It is believed to increase energy and have aphrodisiac qualities. Dong quai, often referred to as "female ginseng," would be a first choice for women. It shares ginseng's invigorating properties and is esteemed as a menstrual cycle normalizer with great utility in menopause as well.

As tonic herbs, both ginseng and dong quai are believed to have a balancing or equalizing effect on mental and physical processes. They are believed to calm hyperactivity and stimulate underactivity in both realms. For older men, saw palmetto may be preferred to ginseng. It is believed to forestall the negative consequences of aging, increases energy, is considered an aphrodisiac, and improves symptoms of prostatic enlargement.

The tonic and hormonal herbs have been added to our regimen because they are beneficial on several levels. By increasing vitality, they have a significant positive effect in the physical sphere. By normalizing reproductive processes and sexual functioning, their effects spill over from physical to emotional and even spiritual realms. If failing self-esteem can be improved, if faltering relationships can be helped, and if intimacy can be fostered or renewed, then many of us would benefit from their usage.

At this point you have, by combining three herbs, formulated a personal herbal mixture that will be beneficial to both mind and body. You have selected from among several herb groups those herbs which best fit your temperament and needs at this time.

Choosing a Final Herb for a Specific Problem

The herbal mixture could well be considered complete at this point. After all, digestion has been promoted, energy and vitality have been advanced, emotional balance has been supported, and sexual function has been improved. On the other hand, many people would now benefit from the addition of a final herb to address a specific problem, a personal health issue or concern. This is what makes your wellness prescription uniquely your own. Rather than cataloging the many choices available, I will instead give you suggestions and guidelines for selection of this final herb.

A reasonable way to begin is to look over the chapter titles of Part Three of this book. Each chapter refers to a major organ system of the body and its associated infirmities. In reviewing this synopsis of medical ailments, you will easily locate any current or chronic problems that are bothering you. For example, you may look up a specific problem in Part Three or the index. Or in browsing through Part Three you may be reminded that you are prone to frequent bladder infections. You could then refer to Chapter 22 and decide that uva ursi should be added to your herbal regimen. Similarly, if you are afflicted with joint pain, the chapter titled "Arthritis" will leap off the page. You will then review Chapter 24 and add an appropriate herb or two to your wellness prescription.

As a final illustration, since this is a prescription for health maintenance, you may choose a fourth herb in the hope of preventing a future difficulty. An example would be a healthy young adult with a strong family history of heart disease. In seeing the chapter title "Cardiovascular Disease," he will be reminded that his father has had a heart attack and two uncles and a grandmother have died of heart failure. He has stopped smoking, watches his diet, and exercises regularly but still wonders whether an herb might be added to his preventive regimen. He may conclude that he would like to add hawthorn or garlic to his regimen.

A second approach is to review the chapter titles in Part Two. Again, the hope is to jog the mind into recognizing continuing problems that could be addressed by an appropriate drug. The chapter title "Diuretics" could serve to remind a young woman that she tends to accumulate fluid at certain times of the month. She would learn in Chapter 11 that horsetail has been beneficially employed in this regard. A cigarette smoker may decide that until he is able to give up this addiction he might want to employ an expectorant so that he could at least help his body in its effort to eliminate cigarette toxins from his lungs. Even better would be to use an expectorant as part of an overall smoking cessation strategy.

Regardless of which of the above approaches you use to locate the herb that will be most beneficial for your particular requirements, remember that the entire process requires that you heed your body's needs. First and foremost you must define the area of bodily malfunction and the goals of herbal therapy most precisely. As mentioned earlier, the more diligent and honest you are in this endeavor, the more likely you will be to formulate a truly advantageous herbal prescription.

In this chapter I have attempted to guide you through the particulars in the process of formulating an herbal wellness prescription. A few general statements will serve to complete our consideration of this most important area.

From a strictly logistic point of view, I prefer the use of extracts for this application. With extracts, you can simply combine the appropriate number of drops of each herb in a small (for example, one-ounce) glass, add water or juice, and drink. Extracts afford the greatest flexibility in determining the dosage of each component of your mixture; you can literally alter each ingredient by a drop at a time, thus customizing your formula to your exact needs. For example, if you feel that you are being overly relaxed, you can cut back on your sedative herb by a drop or two. You may find that you require only a low dose of one particular herb but maximal dose of another. If you find that extracts leave an unpleasant aftertaste, you might have a mint or piece of gum after each dose.

Once again, since the wellness prescription is designed for daily use, always begin by using each component in the lowest dosage range.

Lastly, and of great importance, don't fall in love with your wellness prescription. Always be ready to experiment and modify. Because you are a living, breathing, changing person, view your prescription in the same light. You are not static but constantly in flux. If you are wise, you are always ready to refine and perfect your health.

Physically we are constantly discarding old cells and forming new cells; we are constantly renewing ourselves on the material level. Emotionally and spiritually our outlook changes from day to day; we move forward or we regress but we are never stagnant. As we become more attuned to our body on all levels, we will perceive changes both physically and emotionally. These will call for changes in our wellness prescription, which must be adjusted accordingly.

The most effective wellness prescription is the one that is best suited to our immediate needs and moves us always to the point of balance and harmony. We are, each of us, unique, special, and ever-changing, and we must be constantly aware of our continuing development. If one becomes acutely ill, a specific herb may be temporarily added and another may be deleted or substituted until health has been reestablished. With chronic illness, permanent changes in our personal herbal prescription may be necessary.

Creating a Wellness Lifestyle

*W*e are all aware that smoking is suicidal, seat belts are mandatory, exercise is beneficial, and moderation is of inestimable value. But wellness is about much more than a listing of do's and don'ts. So instead of stating the obvious, I will concentrate on some more primitive notions that may not be as evident but that could well influence health and vitality. Much of what is to follow has been hinted at or discussed earlier in the book, but I believe it will be convenient to summarize these venerable ideas about wellness in a specific chapter. Again, I emphasize that I am simply attempting to highlight certain elements of a meritorious life that appear to be most sorely lacking in our times.

Recognizing that a human is a composite being could, if rediscovered by contemporary society, be of inestimable value. We tend to separate out the physical, mental, and emotional and deny their dynamic and intimate interaction. Many ignore the spiritual altogether. If instead we saw ourselves as multidimensional and recognized that each realm has profound effects on the others, we would come to a new and more accurate understanding of health and disease.

I am not proposing for a moment that we discard science or that we disregard Western advances in our understanding of disease causation. I am, however, recommending that we reexamine the relationship between the emotional and physical and once again give spirituality the status it deserves.

Our physical nature is quite obvious; it can be immediately touched and seen. Our spirituality is often less readily apparent. It is nonetheless unmistakably present in the writings of Shakespeare, the music of Bach, and the cathedrals of Europe. We must recognize our constituent parts and endeavor to nurture and support ourselves on all levels. An afternoon in a museum or a quiet evening of reading may be as important to good health as a jog around the block. A hearty laugh may be even more therapeutic.

Health is achieved and maintained only by sustaining vitality in all spheres. The person who is thriving on all levels is both more re-sistant to the development of disease and better able to fight disease should she become infirm. Concentrating on the physical is not enough. Growing intellectually likewise will not suffice. Only by completing the picture and finding emotional and spiritual balance can optimal health be attained. This is a time-honored notion. To-day it is being voiced by a small but growing number of advocates and is just beginning to be discussed in scientific circles. I hope that this concept will continue to be taken more seriously and will con-tribute much to our understanding of the human condition.

In alternative medical thinking, people are considered largely responsible for their own health. While this includes the usual habits of a healthy lifestyle that we are all aware of, it has more deep-seated implications. It emphasizes the virtue of self-reliance and puts the individual in the position of primacy where health is concerned. This differs dramatically from the common outlook shared by most of our contemporaries. While we may give lip ser-vice to living in a judicious manner, the fact is that few follow such a path, and we all expect the physician to bail us out when the in-evitable health consequences occur. We all know what we should do, but because of the miracles of modern medicine we feel less obliged to do it.

In earlier times we had more modest expectations of our heal-ers. Marvelous cures were not so frequently observed, and diseases often took their inexorable course. Prayer and the spirit realm were often implored in serious cases, thus underlining the desperateness of the situation. In more primitive societies the healer was not asso-ciated with the "quick fix," so it was best to stay healthy and avoid the encounter altogether. Accordingly, what we would now call preventive medicine was a bedrock concept rather than a guilty af-terthought, and self-reliance in health matters was the order of the day. Most common ailments were treated in the home, according to time-honored family traditions.

While we should all certainly avail ourselves of the wonders of modern medicine when indicated, I feel that a certain self-sufficiency may be beneficial. Although certainly it is important to consult the doctor if you are truly ill, not every minor ache and pain requires a visit to the doctor—and viral illnesses do not require antibiotics. Herbalists hold the body and its self-recuperative powers in very high regard. Herbal dogma insists that when illness strikes, the body will mount an appropriate response, and a major function of the healer is to support the body's natural healing imperative. Much of herbal therapeutics is geared toward enhancing bodily processes, thus hastening a cure.

This is not a viewpoint widely held in Western countries. Somewhere in the process of becoming advanced, civilized, sophisticated, and scientific, we have lost touch with simple wisdom. We need to be reminded that prior to modern medicine, people were able to overcome all but the most devastating of diseases on their own. We forget that our body is a constant battleground, with war continually being waged between pathogenic influences that mean us harm and our own intrinsic defenses, which are ever struggling to maintain our health.

The manner in which an invasion of infectious organisms is countered by our own protective forces is a thousand times more complex than any battle plan devised by the most intense of military geniuses. Only now in the laboratory are we beginning to understand the multiple players of our immune system; their complex roles; and the intricate, perfectly timed and executed interplay among them.

Somewhere between the innate wisdom of our ancestors and the specialized understanding of the laboratory scientist, we have forgotten that such wonders occur. We have lost faith in their great effectiveness. We need to recall the grandeur of the human body, respect its capabilities, and realize once again that most cure comes from within and not without. We have spent a better part of a century seeking health "out there"—in the doctor's office, in a hypodermic needle, in a hospital bed. It is time we begin again to look inward, appreciate our body's great potentiality, and work with it rather than against it to achieve maximal wellness.

We must also take stock of the toll that sickness takes on the body. With each successful recovery a battle has been waged and won. But energies are depleted by each encounter with disease. Rest and sufficient convalescence are necessary after each occurrence of illness. Tonic herbs, which have great revitalizing potential, are most important at this time. These simple measures are simply further examples of the respect that ancient cultures have always accorded the human body.

Remember finally that even with the most serious of diseases—even when miracle drugs, surgical procedures, or modern-day heroics have been successfully employed—your body's own inherent ability to rebound and rebuild will determine the ultimate outcome.

From times preceding recorded history to the present era, the primacy of the body must continually be affirmed.

Balance is a bellwether notion in the wisdom of the sages. The Greek physicians balanced the four bodily fluids and temperaments, Indian healers balanced the three humors, and in Chinese medicine yin and yang are the complementary principles.

We understand the necessity of a lifestyle characterized by moderation and symmetry. We have been advised about the benefits of exercise; we are warned to decrease our intake of fats and sugars and replace them with grains, fruits, and vegetables. We know work must be offset by play and exercise by rest. In the emotional sphere, however, modern humanity abhors the very idea of balance. Negative feelings are avoided at any cost, and unpleasant thoughts are cast out like thieves in the night. We desire only to feel good and will go to any extreme to avoid emotional discomfort. Alcohol, drugs, cults, and self-indulgence are simply escape mechanisms from reality.

Alternative wisdom, however, appreciates the necessity of the full range of emotions from the most exhilarating joy to the deepest melancholy. The truly integrated human has experienced the gamut of emotions and is the better for it. There is value in the full range of feelings, and the entire human drama is to be savored. There is dignity to suffering and pain, and some value in even the most apparently senseless of tragedies.

When we are able to accept this worldview, when we begin to feel that we are not the be-all and end-all of creation but rather part of a larger whole, a major step forward will have been taken. When we begin to appreciate the necessity of all that is—good and bad, right and wrong, joy and suffering, birth and death—we will be on the correct path to understanding and truth. And when we can truly celebrate creation and know that we are an essential part of that most inexpressible mystery, then wellness will truly be ours.

Cancer: A Complementary Approach

*O*ne-third of all Americans will develop cancer, which is second only to cardiovascular disease as a cause of death in the United States. Cancer is obviously a most serious disease, and primary treatment rests with the practitioner of scientific medicine. Dependent on the site of the cancer and its extent, medical treatment might consist of surgery, radiation therapy, chemotherapy, or some combination of these.

Herbal therapy, however, may provide the patient with significant palliation or relief of cancer symptoms, and adoption of principles that underlie an herbal lifestyle would also decrease its incidence. Perhaps most importantly, the herbal mindset fosters a degree of harmony and tranquillity that is highly beneficial for the patient struggling with this catastrophic disease.

We are well aware that certain lifestyle factors play a major role in cancer causation. Of greatest significance by far, cigarette smoking accounts for one-third of all male and one-tenth of all female cancer deaths in the United States. Lung cancer, the premier cancer killer, for example, is ten times more common in male smokers than in male nonsmokers. Excessive exposure to sun radiation is the most important risk factor for skin cancer. Pollution of air and water will increasingly contribute to environmentally caused diseases, including cancer.

There is substantial evidence that diet contributes significantly to cancers of many sites and that significant inroads would be made by following a few simple recommendations. These include reduction of fat intake; increased consumption of fruits, vegetables, and grains; and reduction in consumption of alcohol, salt-cured, and smoked foods. A detailed discussion of all factors that contribute to the development of cancer is not practical here.

I have demonstrated that ancient medical thinking, millennia old, conforms with the newest concepts of the genesis of cancer and that we today have no monopoly on wisdom. The ancient sages who proposed a healthy balanced diet, moderation in all things, harmony with and respect for nature, and individual responsibility for our own health could make their points with equal validity today. Twentieth-century science simply validates what was, for our ancestors, intuitive knowledge.

Several herbs have been used to fight cancer. Astragalus has been used extensively in China, and its anticancerous effect is believed to be due to its ability to boost immune function. A tumor-inhibiting principle has been isolated by the USDA in echinacea, so that this drug also has anticancer effects mediated via immune mechanisms (Figure 34, #1).

The tonic herbs licorice and ginseng have also developed a reputation as advantageous in cancer treatment (Figure 34, #2), but echinacea and astragalus should really be considered first-line herbs, more in tune with current thinking about tumor biology. *Remember that scientific medicine however should always have primacy in cancer therapy.*

Significant palliation of symptoms of cancer can be afforded by appropriate and timely herbal therapy. Formulation of an herbal mixture for cancer patients would follow guidelines quite similar to those for HIV, and many helpful hints will be found in Chapter 35.

A digestive herb would always be called for in cancer patients because nutritional status must always be supported and vital energy maximized. Cardamom could certainly be employed, but particular symptoms may warrant consideration of another digestive. The reader is referred to the Chapters 7 and 8 for a more thorough discussion of the aromatic and bitter digestive herbs.

Nausea and vomiting secondary to the disease itself or treatment (chemotherapy or radiotherapy) may respond to ginger or peppermint. Diarrhea can be controlled with cinnamon, ginger, or hops. More detailed consideration of these subjects is found in Chapter 23 on gastrointestinal disorders. Because cancer can affect all organ

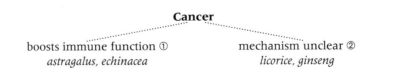

Cancer

boosts immune function ①
astragalus, echinacea

mechanism unclear ②
licorice, ginseng

FIGURE 34

systems, the appropriate herb to allay symptoms in each individual case may be found in appropriate chapters in this book.

Finally, an herb to increase energy is of value in virtually all patients with cancer. Fenugreek or saw palmetto may be employed early on, while dong quai may be a more judicious choice in late stage disease.

Dealing with our own mortality is never easy. It represents, for all of us, the last great task of life. Many of us deny our mortality until the last possible moment and then react with fear and rage. Myriad popular books, on the other hand, promise that death is but a return to the light and the beginning of an eternity of peace and bliss. We each must choose our own particular worldview, and the decision is a profoundly personal one.

The process of dying, however, is less individual and for most of us follows a well-defined sequence. Stages of grief are passed through in an almost predictable fashion. These are considered most thoroughly and sensitively in the writings of Dr. Elisabeth Kübler-Ross, and I recommend her work most wholeheartedly. Anger, denial, depression: the specter of death will call forth the strongest of emotional responses. The patient must work through a minefield of conflicting feelings, and the passage requires all of one's strength and maturity. I am not suggesting that this ultimate journey is ever easy, but it can be made easier.

In ancient cultures, the cycle of life is respected. In early agricultural societies, people experienced the seasons much more personally than we do today. Their existence depended on the palpable realities of the crop cycle: germination, growth, and eventual death. People's sensibilities were attuned to the undeniable reality of death and rebirth. Their mythology and religion reflected these insights, and their own place in this grand scheme was accepted.

In our age of scientific medicine, we exert great effort in an attempt to outsmart nature and outwit death. While this is a most praiseworthy pursuit, its concomitant mental outlook is defiance toward and contempt of death. Such a mindset may not be so beneficial. When faced with a terminal illness, resignation and peaceful acceptance may represent true mental health even today.

Traditionally people have always placed great stock in family and friends. In primitive times there was great allegiance to the tribe, from which each member derived great strength. When someone is faced with terminal illness, loved ones can provide great solace and comfort.

This is not the time to be taken from family and friends—to be deposited in a cold, impersonal institution. Rather, the pillows should be fluffed up, the patient tucked in his own bed. Family and friends should be called together. Reminiscence, laughter, and even a few tears are called for now. Honest emotions, sensitivity, affection, and genuine caring are the only medications that are absolutely required. The undeniable healing that occurs will be experienced by all present.

Complementary Medicine: HIV as Model

*T*his chapter gives readers a practical application of much of what has been discussed in this book. I have chosen to use HIV infection as an illustrative example because of its obvious clinical importance and widespread current interest. However, you don't have to have AIDS or be at high risk for developing it to gain a great deal from this chapter, because the principles are applicable to all infections. I also have a particular interest in this illness because in one of my roles (I am the medical director of a clinic for drug addicts) many of my patients do have HIV disease.

HIV and AIDS represent the polarities of human infection with a transmittable virus. When a person is HIV positive, that means only that a person has been infected with the human immunodeficiency virus (HIV) and harbors that virus within specific immune cells in the body. The patient has no discernible symptoms at this stage.

In most cases, the passage of time results in a progressive destruction of increasing numbers of the infected immune cells (T cells). The method of immune cell destruction by the HIV virus is not under-stood with certainty at this time, but clearly some trigger activates the virus, causing massive viral reproduction which results in disruption of T cells.

When the number of T cells reaches a critical low level, the patient begins manifesting symptoms. Once symptoms develop, a diagnosis of AIDS (acquired immunodeficiency syndrome) is made. These symptoms are primarily caused by infection with microorganisms that generally do not cause disease in healthy individuals (opportunistic infections) but can cause devastating illness in patients with an impaired immunity. Thus the spectrum of HIV ranges from the asymptomatic carrier state, through a stage of symptomatic infections, ultimately leading to a life-threatening illness.

HIV infection absolutely requires all the best that modern medicine has to offer. From the earliest asymptomatic stage, the infected individual needs to be followed at regular intervals by his primary care physician. However, it is my firm conviction that likewise, from the onset, aspects of alternative medical thinking can be beneficially employed.

The first stage of infection, when the patient is HIV positive but exhibits no symptoms, is a long period of an average of eight years or more. While modern medicine has nothing to offer the patient at this stage, it is nonetheless a critical time period for two reasons. First, the patient, though feeling perfectly well, is fully infectious at this time, and therefore appropriate precautions must be taken to protect sexual partners. Additionally, those with an ancient medical perspective would view this period as a "window of opportunity." The hope at this early stage would be to stave off the full-blown disease for as long as possible and to enhance the body's defenses so that when AIDS does manifest itself, the patient is at maximum possible vitality. For these reasons, I strongly recommend periodic screening tests for HIV exposure in high-risk groups so that diagnosis can be made as early as possible.

There are no scientific studies clearly demonstrating that employing a restorative alternative medical regimen either prolongs latency or stimulates immunity in infected patients, but anecdotal evidence increasingly supports these contentions. It has been demonstrated that the simple hygienic measure of smoking cessation prolongs life expectancy in patients with HIV. I think it is simply a logical progression to feel reasonably sure that other healthful measures will favorably influence the outcome in HIV positive patients. I will highlight some aspects of a complementary approach in the following paragraphs.

In alternative medicine, each of us is considered responsible for our own health. There is a growing sense among more holistic medical practitioners that the simple act of taking charge and assuming responsibility for our own well-being has a major positive therapeutic effect.

Additionally, in ancient medical systems, how we choose to live in times of good health is considered an important determinant of what transpires when illness supervenes. Thus the asymptomatic HIV positive patient, most especially, should follow an advantageous lifestyle known to foster wellness. Even the simplest matters should not be overlooked.

Diet should be nutritious. Raw fruits and vegetables are considered restorative in summer, while hearty stews and soups are considered therapeutic in winter. One should choose fresh and unadulterated foods over those with preservatives and additives. Caffeine, alcohol, fats, and refined carbohydrates should be avoided. Caloric intake should be geared to maintenance of ideal body weight.

Exercise provides a variety of benefits. It increases levels of natural opiatelike chemicals (endorphins) in the brain that nurture a positive outlook. Regular exercise will prevent a buildup of excess nervous energy and anxiety, encouraging a stable emotional state and enhancing the quality of sleep. It increases muscle strength and the personal feeling of vitality.

Rest likewise is a cornerstone and most important principle in maximizing energy. Herbalists believe that a short period of rest is often sufficient to tip the balance and reverse a nagging condition. Similarly, sufficient periods of quiet relaxation and untroubled sleep are essential in maintaining the body's dominance over the HIV during the asymptomatic period.

Your body will tell you when rest is necessary and you must be attentive to it. A person infected with HIV will need more sleep than before. Increasing one's rest periods must not be considered as a concession to the virus; rather it must be viewed as part of an overall strategy to hold it at bay.

A simple but significant point needs to be made here. It may be argued that the modern physician would find no fault with any of the above. Although it is undeniably true that no M.D. would argue against an adequate diet, regular exercise, and sufficient rest, the reality is that few would consider these as central to a therapeutic regimen. Too many physicians concentrate on side effects of medications, possible symptoms of opportunistic infections, and changes in T-cell counts while overlooking the importance of basic self-care.

These notions, while not essential in the modern view of health, are however at the foundation of the alternative medical paradigm. In this view, the body has its own inherent healing tendencies. The simple measures above represent an opportunity to enhance the body's own curative powers by physical means.

Enhancement must also occur on other levels as well. A growing appreciation of beauty and the arts must be fostered. The intellect must be stimulated and the emotions nourished. Caring relationships and the full expression of loving and sharing become essential components of a healing formula. Spirituality must be nurtured, and a sense of harmony and peace should be encouraged.

Healing is accomplished by a balancing of all areas of human life into a harmonious whole. Health is achieved by maximizing vitality in all spheres—mental, emotional, physical, and spiritual. While the scientist may give lip service to this approach, the ancient healer considers it the bedrock of true wellness.

These are the general reinvigorating measures suggested by an application of principles common to alternative medicine. While less dramatic than genetically engineered medications, laser-beam radiation therapy, and life-saving emergency surgery, their significance must not be downplayed. But, in addition to these broadly applicable precepts, more specific strategies can be employed in an alternative medical regimen.

An advantageous herbal prescription can be developed by utilizing the approach outlined in Chapter 32. As always, it is recommended that one begin by selecting an herb that will aid in digestive processes, thus affording the body maximum nutritional energy. As a general rule, the aromatic digestives would be favored in this setting, and cardamom would be particularly well suited, but the patient is advised to review appropriate sections before making a selection.

The bitter digestives are certainly not contraindicated and can be considered for use if warranted by the clinical state. For example, in the setting of drug abuse, milk thistle would be a prime candidate because of its beneficial effects on the liver. In any case the foundation of any restorative prescription should be a digestive herb.

Infestation with the HIV virus is naturally cause for concern, and even the most stoic of HIV positive patients will at times exhibit symptoms of anxiety or apprehension. Valerian is an excellent natural tranquilizer and can be employed to good effect here. Since it is nonsedating it has no adverse effect on physical prowess or mental acuity. It is a mild herb that will not sap the body's resources when used appropriately. For most patients occasional use when warranted will suffice. Those patients who suffer a constant, vague sense of apprehension or restlessness may require a small dose as part of a daily regimen in order to achieve emotional balance. The other sedative herbs are likewise of service, and the reader is again advised to review the appropriate segments of the book. Ginseng (perhaps more for men) or dong quai (generally recommended for women) may be added for their overall balancing effect, helping to promote equilibrium on the mental and physical levels. Both increase vitality, a most important consideration in this setting.

We have, at this point, combined several herbs that will be broadly beneficial in the fight against HIV. They will increase availability of nutritional energy, help calm those who are tense or ill at ease, nudge the patient toward physical and mental balance, and increase overall vigor. Now we will add two herbs that are specifically believed to benefit immune function.

Astragalus is a tonic herb believed to be specifically fortifying to the immune system. Since it shares many of the properties of ginseng and dong quai as listed above, it can either be substituted for these or simply added to a mixture to increase their effectiveness. Astragalus and ginseng, in fact, are frequently combined in ancient Chinese medicine, since ginseng is believed to promote attacking energy, while astragalus is believed to both increase bodily defenses and boost immune function. In Western herbal tradition, astragalus is frequently used with echinacea, a powerful immune stimulant.

The specific triad of ginseng, astragalus, and echinacea would appear to be a fitting combination in the setting of HIV disease, maximally stimulating immune function, fostering vitality and balance, and incorporating both Chinese and Western herbal traditions. By systematically applying the principles advanced in Chapter 32 we have put together an herbal mixture that could well benefit patients in the asymptomatic stage of HIV infection.

Many practitioners and proponents of complementary medicine are advocates of vitamin therapy as well, and supplementation with these vital substances may likewise be profitable. The incorporation of additional vitamins to a sound herbal and dietary regimen is especially encouraged at this asymptomatic stage. I have not given recommendations on vitamin therapy for other maladies since it is well beyond the scope of this book. Such information is readily available elsewhere. My goal here is simply to demonstrate that vitamin therapy can well be, and often is, included in a complementary framework. Let me give a concrete example.

Patients with borderline levels of pantothenic acid demonstrate decreased resistance to infection, so the addition of 10 milligrams per day of this vitamin seems judicious. The entire vitamin B group, in fact, has been associated with improved immune function, so a high-potency vitamin B complex supplement is recommended.

Vitamin E is linked to augmented immune response, and I would suggest a dose of 400 milligrams a day of mixed tocopherols. Zinc is indispensable for normal functioning of the body's protective defenses, and a 10-milligram supplement taken daily can only be beneficial. As a reasonable approach to vitamin supplementation in

HIV, I would therefore recommend a high-potency B complex per-haps with additional pantothenic acid, along with vitamin E and zinc in order to maintain and enhance immune function.

The above combination of general measures, herbal therapy, and vitamin therapy represent for me a sound approach to the difficult problem of asymptomatic HIV disease. I feel that it is imperative to emphasize that this approach simply seems to make good sense to one particular scientifically trained physician with an interest in herbal-ism, complementary medicine, and mind-body interactions. It is but one of a great number of approaches that might be employed in this situation.

I stress that no scientific controlled studies have demonstrated the efficacy of this particular model and that it has received no offi-cial sanction or approval. Yet I will say, if without proof yet equally without hesitation, that I feel that patients will genuinely benefit from the overall strategy being recommended.

Throughout the asymptomatic phase, it is assumed that the patient has maintained regular contact with his primary care physi-cian. As disease progresses and symptoms become prominent, the role of scientific medicine assumes greater import. Disease progres-sion and the development of opportunistic infection correlate roughly with decreasing numbers of T cells destroyed by the virus. Often when T cell counts fall to about 500 cells per microliter, minor in-fections begin to occur.

This early symptomatic stage has been termed ARC (AIDS-related complex) and is considered an indication for antiviral therapy. At this time, Zidovudine (AZT) is the preferred antiviral treatment for patients with T cell counts under 500. AZT therapy has been demon-strated in clinical trials to be effective on the basis of delaying progression to advanced disease, fewer deaths, fewer opportunistic infections, and increasing T cell counts.

When T cells drop below 200, prophylactic antibiotic therapy to prevent *P. carinii* pneumonia (PCP), a major cause of death in AIDS, is often given in addition to AZT. Progression to advanced AIDS is heralded by the appearance of more severe infections, often associ-ated with constitutional symptoms. These signs of generalized disease include fever, involuntary weight loss, or unexplained diarrhea.

The overall management of patients who have symptomatic HIV disease should be entrusted to the scientific physician. Only she will be able to correctly diagnose the opportunistic infections as they occur, and choose appropriate therapy administered either at home or in the hospital. Standard medical textbooks may be referred to by those interested in the most up-to-date treatment of symptomatic HIV. My purpose here is not to catalog modern medicine's treatment of AIDS, but simply to underscore its importance.

Patients with progressive HIV should not forsake the herbal regimen recommended for those who are asymptomatic. In addition, herbal medications may be added for specific problems that may become troubling but do not require prescription drugs. Minor nausea, diarrhea, throat irritation, and other lesser symptoms may, with your physician's approval, be treated in this manner.

A restorative program, as developed and described above, is perhaps even more important at this stage of advancing disease than in the latent stage of illness. Strict adherence to an herbal regimen, maintenance of adequate food intake, and measures to ensure continued emotional and spiritual growth are essential aspects of a strategy of revival. While false hope is to be discouraged, one should nurture a sense of quiet confidence and a genuine appreciation for life and its continuous renewal.

I am a firm believer in the value of alternative medicine, the benefits of herbal therapy, and the extraordinary untapped potential of a balanced and harmonious lifestyle. I consider these the cornerstone of good health and the most basic prescription for a life of wellness. These are the ideas I try to nurture in my patients, and I see the benefits daily in my practice. Indeed, much of this book has been written to support these concepts.

However, if there is a single creed to which I must wholeheartedly assent, it is that such a system sometimes needs to be supplemented. I choose this word carefully. By invoking scientific medicine when needed, those of us who believe in herbal therapy do not deny our belief in alternative medicine or its corollary lifestyle. We respect the ancient heritage that has afforded us such great benefit. But we recognize that it, like all things human, has limitations. While steadfastly adhering to our alternative beliefs, we invite sympathetic physicians, armed with science and technology, to supplement our foundation.

Despite the widespread beliefs and prejudices of their practitioners, alternative and scientific medicine are not mutually exclusive. Neither has a monopoly on truth. Each is brimming with validity and vitality. Most importantly, each would be strengthened by an alliance with the other. Each is a part of the whole. One, in short, complements the other. There is a place where alternative and scientific medicine must interface. If the physicians, acupuncturists, and herbalists cannot find that spot, maybe the patients will have to point it out.

CONCLUSION

I was recently in the medical library at the hospital and I saw a brand-new edition (the thirteenth) of *Harrison's Principles of Internal Medicine*. I recalled how we doctors-in-training eagerly awaited the publication of updated volumes of this scholarly work and recalled that my first issue was of the sixth edition. I have been buying updated versions periodically since then and reminded myself to order a copy when I got to the office.

It was difficult for me to accept that I have been a physician now through over half of the editions of Harrison, yet the fact was indisputable. I tried to disregard the powerful wave of nostalgia that overtook me and began to peruse this venerable textbook.

Unchanged was the old familiar format that has served me so well both in training and in my continuing years in practice. The "Introduction to Clinical Medicine" and "Cardinal Manifestations of Disease" were read with great diligence, and even greater pride, by generations of medical students as they made the transition from lecture halls to the wards. These sections were there, as always, to enlighten and motivate.

Unconsciously I felt a great respect for my profession, its grand purpose, and its most esteemed practitioners. My mind wandered to those professors who most inspired and guided me and the healing work done by so many whom I would never meet but know only through their work and reputation. It is a very humbling experience to consider that you share the same calling as men and women named Pasteur, Curie, and Salk.

I recalled the many sleepless nights spent with critically ill patients, the heroic measures we often employed, and the excruciating decisions to sometimes discontinue them. I remember some patients who made it and some who did not. Especially those who did not.

I recollected how deeply it all affected us, and how we were expected to be passive and composed in consoling the loved ones when all we could do was not quite enough. I recalled comforting nurses before such encounters; I also remembered being comforted. Health and disease, living and dying all can become a pretty dirty business at times, and criticism is always easy for those on the outside, but I couldn't help but be reminded that there is unquestioned nobility about the whole endeavor.

By far the longest chapter in the thirteenth edition of Harrison was not present in the sixth edition. You see, the disease it describes was not known when I was a medical student. The chapter is entitled "Human Immunodeficiency Virus (HIV) Disease: AIDS and Related Disorders." Times surely have changed but not always for the better.

The book is much thicker now, and the printing is smaller. Knowledge continues to accumulate at a staggering rate. One has to appreciate the extraordinary amount of dedication that goes into ensuring that stagnation does not occur, that new information and understanding are continuously forthcoming, and that new treatments and cures reliably get to the patients.

All this occurs, for the most part unheralded, in the laboratories and on the wards of our teaching hospitals and research institutions. The most promising results are reported in the medical literature. Harrison's textbook is a marvelous encyclopedic summary of all that is state-of-the-art in modern medicine. It encapsulates the greatest advances that scientific medicine has effected, and as such it is truly awe-inspiring. For a moment I believed that perhaps I have been a bit unfair in the way I have represented my own vocation of scientific medicine in this book. Therefore I will here and now affirm unequivocally my respect and admiration for this exalted calling. It has served humankind extremely well, and I am genuinely honored to be a practitioner. If other human pursuits had been done with half the diligence and a fraction of the devotion, we would all be living in a far better world.

Yet, while wandering through the index before closing the book, I could not help but note the omissions. Nothing on herbs or acupuncture. No citation for alternative or complementary medicine. No mention of mind-body interactions or therapeutic touch. No meditation or spirituality.

Maybe that is how it should be. These are not scientific notions and perhaps should not be included in a scientific textbook.

But it is my deep conviction that they are healing notions. And that is why this book was written.

EPILOGUE

Knowing one's limitations is perhaps the beginning of wisdom. Having completed this book, you should be ready to apply what you have learned in an orderly and considered manner. Begin prudently, treat only the most nonthreatening conditions, and expect modest results. In this way you can only be pleasantly surprised.

As you gain experience and confidence in the use of herbs, the range of conditions you will comfortably treat will expand, and the results will be even more rewarding. If you ever are in doubt, do not hesitate to seek professional advice.

Always keep in mind your own responsibility for your own health, and never neglect the simple and most obvious. Work must be balanced by play, exercise by rest. The spiritual and emotional realms cannot be sacrificed for the physical and mental. Meditation and contemplation are essential to total wellness. Any life that neglects these spheres is incomplete and by its very nature unhealthy.

It is my deeply held contention that scientific and herbal methods of healing are complementary. In some situations speed and strength are of life-and-death import while in others grace and delicacy are favored. By listening to your own body you will usually know intuitively which approach is called for.

Thus, while both herbal and scientific medicine are limited in applicability, together they constitute a whole. Accordingly, knowing the limitations of each approach is the beginning of true medical wisdom. Not surprisingly, the patients are further along in this understanding than most of their doctors.

REFERENCES

General References

Balch, James F. and Phyllis A. *Prescription for Nutritional Healing.* Garden City Park, New York: Avery Publishing Group, Inc., 1990.

Lust, John. *The Herb Book.* New York: Bantam Books, 1994.

Mills, Simon. *Out of the Earth: The Science and Practice of Herbal Medicine.* Viking/Penguin, 1992.

Mindell, Earl. *Earl Mindell's Herb Bible.* New York: Simon and Schuster/Fireside, 1992.

Mowrey, Daniel B. *Herbal Tonic Therapies.* New Canaan, CT: Keats Publishing, Inc., 1993.

Polunin, Miriam, and Christopher Robbins. *The Natural Pharmacy: An Illustrated Guide to Natural Medicine.* New York: Collier Books, 1992.

Chapter References

Chapter 1

Cousins, Norman. *Anatomy of an Illness as Perceived by the Patient.* New York, London: W. W. Norton and Company, 1979.

Ecclesiastes 3:1.

Moyers, Bill. *Healing and the Mind.* New York: Doubleday, 1995.

Chapter 2

Bickell, William H. et al. "Immediate versus delayed fluid resuscitation for hypotensive patients with penetrating torso injuries." *New England Journal of Medicine* vol. 331 (October 27, 1994): 1105–1109.

Chapter 8

Faber, K. "Der loewenzahn = taraxacum officinale weber." *Pharmazie* 13, no. 7 (1958): 423–435.

Glatzel, H., and Hackenberg, K. "Roentgenological studies of the effects of the effects of bitters on digestive organs." *Planta Medica* vol. 1583 (1967): 223–232.

Chapter 9

Foster, Steven. "Feverfew: heading up herbal reliefs," *Better Nutrition for Today's Living* 57, no. 5 (May 1995): 74.

Galley, P., and N. Sofi. "Tanakan et cerveau senile. Etude radis circulo-graphique." *Bordeaux Med.* 171 (1977).

Chapter 10

Della Loggia, R., et al. "Depressive effect of *chamomilla recutita* (l.) rausch, tubular flowers on central nervous system in mice." *Pharm. Res. Comm.* 14, no. 2 (1982), 153–162.

Shipochliev, T. "Pharmacological study of several essential oils. I. Effects on the smooth muscle." *Vet. Med.* (Prague) 13, nos. 8–9 (1968), 64–69.

Chapter 13

Stimpel, M., A. Proksch, et al. "Macrophage activation and induction of macrophage cytotoxicity by purified polysaccharide fractions from the plant *Echinacea purpurea.*" *Infection and Immunity* 46, no. 3 (1984): 845–849.

Chapter 14

Mukerji, B. *Indian Pharmaceutical Codex.* New Delhi, India: 1953, p. 60.

Nasyrov, K. M., and D. N. Lazareva. "Study of the anti-inflammatory activity of glycyrrhizin acid derivatives." *Farmak-i Toksikol* 43, no. 4 (1980): 399–404.

Yoshiro, K. "The physiological actions of tang-kuai and onidium. *Bull Oriental Healing Arts Inst.* 10 (1985): 267–78.

Chapter 16

Crimi A., and A. Russo. "Extract of S*erenoa repens* for the treatment of the functional disturbances of prostate hypertrophy." *Med Praxis* 4 (1983): 47–51.

Chapter 20

Allegra C., G. Pollari, A. Criscuolo, et. al. "*Centella asiatica* extract in venous disorders of the lower limbs, comparative clinico-instrumental studies with a placebo." *Clin Terap* 99, (1981): 507–13.

Petkov, V. "Plants with hypotensive, antiatheromatous, and coronary dilating action." *American Journal of Chinese Medicine* 7, (1979): 197–236.

Chapter 26

Klich, R., and B. Gladback. "Verhaltensstoerungen im kindsalter und deren therapie." *Medezinische Welt,* 26, no. 25 (1975), 1252–1254.

Chapter 34

Kübler-Ross, Elisabeth. *On Death and Dying.* New York: Macmillan, 1969.

Chapter 36

Isselbacher, Karl J. et al., editors. *Harrison's Principles of Internal Medicine, 13th Edition.* New York: McGraw-Hill, 1994.

INDEX

Abdominal pain, cinnamon for, 36
Absinthe, 37
Acid reflux and peppermint, 47
Acne: burdock for, 75, 118; echinacea for, 55, 75, 118; nettle for, 76, 118
Acquired immunodeficiency syndrome. *See* AIDS
Acupuncture, xvi, xviii, 7, 8, 20, 126, 150, 152
Acute illnesses, 33
Aerobic exercise, 23
Africa, 54
Aftertaste, 133
Aging, 91, 115, 116, 117; and ginseng, 60, 78, 116; and male hormonal herbs, 62–63, 116; and saw palmetto, 63, 79, 116; and seven barks, 62, 79, 116
Agitation, 105
AIDS, xii, xiii, 33, 148–149, 152; echinacea for, 55; prophylactic antibiotic therapy for, 148. *See also* HIV
AIDS-related complex (ARC), 148
Alcohol, 24, 95, 138, 139, 145; additive effects, 45, 106; and high blood pressure, 85; and liver disease, 128
Aldosterone and licorice, 58
Allantoin and comfrey, 67
Allergies, 87, 88, 89
Aloe, 66, 80
Alternative medicine, xii, xvii–xviii, 126, 136, 152; and HIV, 144, 146, 149–150; physical, mental, emotional, and

spiritual levels, 56; section of National Institutes of Health, xv; versus scientific medicine, xvi, 12–16, 93. *See also* Complementary medicine; Herbal medicine; Scientific medicine
American Cancer Society, 61
American Indians, 6, 18, 21, 55, 64, 66, 113
American Journal of Chinese Medicine, 48
Americas and herbalism, 6
Amino acids, xi
Ancient religion: and death, 141; and herbal medicine, 5–6
Ancient societies, xv, 3, 4, 7, 18, 56, 140, 141, 144
Angelica, 19, 36, 51, 68, 87, 88, 94, 96, 97, 98, 128
Anger, 8, 141
Angina, 83
Angioplasties, xiii
Antiaging. *See* Aging
Antibacterial properties: of elecampane, 50, 74; of thyme, 50, 74
Antibiotics, 4, 18, 41, 82, 89, 115, 120, 121, 136; in AIDS treatment, 148; for urinary tract infections, 92
Antifungal properties of thyme, 50
Anti-inflammatory properties, 53; of cayenne, 42; of dandelion, 39; of feverfew, 43, 100; of gentian, 39; of licorice, 58
Antiseptic properties: of devil's claw, 54; of echinacea, 55, 120, 121; of uva ursi, 49